A WOMAN'S GUIDE TO CONFRONTING, DIAGNOSING, AND TREATING SEXUAL PAIN

HEALING PAINFUL SEX

DEBORAH COADY, MD,
& NANCY FISH, MSW, MPH

SEAL PRESS

PRAISE FOR *HEALING PAINFUL SEX*

"A concise, clear, and comprehensive resource that informs and empowers women to get the care they deserve. Coady and Fish tend to women's bodies, minds, and relationships, illustrating precisely the type of integrated and holistic treatment approach that stands the best chance of success."

—Marta Meana, PhD, author of *Obesity Surgery:*
Stories of Altered Lives

"*Healing Painful Sex* identifies many of the mysteries behind diagnoses women commonly receive, and offers solutions to various conditions and disorders. This book makes it easy to understand challenging diagnoses. I highly recommend it to women and their healthcare providers."

—Amy Stein, PT, MPT, BCB-PMD, author of *Heal Pelvic Pain* and
Founder of Beyond Basics Physical Therapy, New York

"Sexual pain loses its mystery in a book that comprehensively covers the myriad physical causes and treatments available to replace misdiagnosis and improper treatment. For women, here is hope that cuts through the murkiness of vulvodynia to clear diagnosis for vulvar pain."

—Elizabeth G. Stewart, MD, author, *The V Book*

"This book offers thoughtful, often holistic and spiritual advice reminiscent of Eastern Medicine. Anatomical terms and biology are demystified to form the basis of therapy. Great emphasis is placed on listening to the patient and doing a careful, gentle physical examination. Therapy includes physical modalities, medicinal approaches that include both oral and topical drugs, and, when necessary, surgery. I recommend this book enthusiastically to women in search of healing from painful sex."

—A. Lee Dellon, MD, PhD, Professor of Plastic Surgery
and Neurosurgery, Johns Hopkins University

Healing Painful Sex
A Woman's Guide to Confronting, Diagnosing, and Treating Sexual Pain
Copyright © 2011 by Deborah Coady, MD, and Nancy Fish, MSW, MPH

Published by
Seal Press
A Member of the Perseus Books Group
1700 Fourth Street
Berkeley, California

Library of Congress Cataloging-in-Publication Data

Coady, Deborah.
  Healing painful sex : a woman's guide to confronting, diagnosing, and treating sexual pain /
Deborah Coady and Nancy Fish.
      p. cm.
   Summary: "This book is the product of our passionate belief that all women with pelvic pain
need both physical and emotional support"-- Provided by publisher.
  Includes bibliographical references and index.
  ISBN 978-1-58005-363-1 (pbk.)
  1. Dyspareunia. 2. Pelvic pain. I. Fish, Nancy. II. Title.
  RC560.D97C63 2011
  616.85'83--dc23
                                   2011021350

9 8 7 6 5 4 3 2 1

Interior illustrations by Arielle Marks
Interior design by www.meganjonesdesign.com
Printed in the United States of America
Distributed by Publishers Group West

CONTENTS

INTRODUCTION

....

YOU ARE

NOT

ALONE

Learning is the first step in making positive changes within yourself.

—THE DALAI LAMA

I F YOU HAVE ever felt pain during or because of sex, you are not alone.

It's estimated that 16 to 20 percent of all women have had sexual pain at some point in their lives—that's one in every five or six women. Compare that with the percentage of adults (men and women combined) who have asthma (7.7 percent), cancer (8.2 percent), or heart disease (12 percent), and you'll see how shockingly common sexual pain is.

If sexual pain is more common than asthma, cancer, and heart disease, why do we often feel so alone with it? Probably because—unlike asthma, cancer, and heart disease—sexual pain is hard to talk about, even with a doctor. Most women reveal their condition only to a trusted few, and many women feel they can't tell anybody, not even their partners. Most doctors—even the most enlightened gynecologists—are not experienced in treating sexual pain, and they too are often very uncomfortable discussing the subject.

Talking about sexual pain with your doctor can sometimes make you feel even worse than keeping silent. If you've tried to speak with a physician about your condition, you may already have been told—perhaps several times—that your problem is "all in your head," that it stems from your bad attitude toward sex, or that there's nothing that can be done to help you.

We're here to tell you that none of that is true. Sexual pain is almost always caused by an identifiable, verifiable medical condition; it can be treated; and it is not in your head. Very few doctors understand what needs to be done, so help may be hard to find. You may already have been to several doctors, and in your search for effective treatment, you may still have to visit up to a dozen more.

Yes, it is just that difficult to find a physician who is either educated about sexual pain or willing to become so. But help is out there, treatments do exist, and once you find the right person to work with, you have enormous reason for hope. Please don't give up on yourself and your sex life, because we promise you, something can be done.

A full and complete recovery is often possible. In many cases, although you may face some recurring flare-ups of your condition, you can look forward to long periods with no pain or only minimal discomfort. Even in the most difficult situations, you can experience a significant reduction in your pain and can find help for reintroducing sex as a joyous and nourishing part of your life. We promise: Things can get better.

Why are we so sure? Our own experience is our evidence.

ABOUT US

In the rest of this book, we'll be writing with one voice. But for now, let us speak to you individually and personally, so that you can hear each of our stories.

About Nancy

My name is Nancy Fish. I'm a licensed certified social worker with a master's degree in public health, and my training is eclectic. I use a psychodynamic, family-therapy, and cognitive–behavioral approach, and I specialize in chronic illness and grief issues.

When I began my practice fifteen years ago, I never dreamed I would be dealing with my own personal chronic illness—severe pelvic pain so intense that it sometimes seemed to take over the very core of my identity. I went from one specialist to another—seven in all—before I finally found Deborah in 2006.

I'll be honest: When I first walked into Deborah's office, I didn't have much faith that she could help me. But after she spent about two hours with me, her warmth, compassion, and positive attitude gave me hope after being hopeless for so long.

Even though Deborah had years of experience treating women with sexual pain, it took her a while to figure out all the complexities of my condition. Like most women suffering from sexual pain, I did not have one single, simple condition, but a mix of several, and because I'd had inadequate treatment for so long, my conditions had compounded and spread. Deborah made it clear that I would need plenty of patience and fortitude for the journey to healing—but she also promised me that we would get there.

I am still a work in progress, and my treatment continues. But I continue to live happily with my husband, to care for my children, and to engage fully in my work as a therapist. A full and satisfying life is possible for me—but only because I got the treatment that Deborah could provide. In many ways, she saved my life, because I'm not sure how I would have continued had I found no relief from the agonizing pain. Deborah never gave up on me—and she insisted that I never give up on myself. Now that my practice includes many women with sexual pain as well, I try to offer them the same message: Don't lose hope, never give up on living a life with minimal or no pain, and keep believing in your right to enjoy sex and to live a fulfilling life. The reason I'm writing this book is to share that message.

About Deborah

I am Deborah Coady, MD, a board-certified gynecologist who has developed a practice treating women with sexual pain. I didn't intend to make that my focus. But I saw so many women suffering from horrendously painful and complicated vulvovaginal conditions, and I began to see that almost no other doctor understood how to help them. I took it upon myself to fill the gap. I began a process of self-education and carved out a niche in this area of medicine.

Now, although I see women of all kinds, most of my practice time and energy are given to treating women with sexual pain. I'm continually reading, corresponding with colleagues, and attending conferences, making sure to keep up with the latest research developments and the newest treatments. I'm a firm believer in the team approach, and I've developed close relationships with many cherished colleagues in neurology, dermatology, orthopedics, pain management, physiatry, gastroenterology, urology, peripheral nerve surgery, and physical therapy—as well as strong partnerships with Nancy and other therapists. I've come to see that therapy and psychological support are crucial for sexual healing, and I'm happy to promote a holistic approach in this book—focusing on medical treatments, yes, but including advice on nutrition and lifestyle, and emotional support as well.

Before they come to me, most of my patients have already seen several other physicians, and I continue to be shocked at the horror stories I hear, and at the level of misinformation and insensitivity present in what should be a healing community of medicine. I'm grateful to be able to help the women who have been failed by so many other doctors—and I'm fortunate to be able to share my knowledge in this book.

About Our Partnership

After a few months of a solely doctor/patient relationship, we realized how much we have in common professionally. Both of us are committed to validating our patients' concerns and never letting them lose hope. Both of us communicate compassion and empathy, and we understand that women with this difficult condition need to find within themselves an extraordinary degree of fortitude and endurance. The writing of this book fulfilled our mission of helping women do just that.

HOW TO USE THIS BOOK

This book is the product of our passionate belief that all women with sexual pain need both physical and emotional support. Our goal is to help you understand:

- what is causing your pain;
- how to navigate a complicated medical system;
- how to treat your pain;
- how to cope with your emotions;
- how to deal with your family and friends; and
- how to move on to a fulfilling life.

We begin, in Part 1, with "Naming the Problem." We believe that isolation is deadly—especially for the intense experience of sexual pain. Chapter 1 will help you find ways to share your situation with one or two people who can help you make medical decisions and work through the emotions that inevitably arise.

In Chapter 2, we move on to doctors. Many of our patients have had horrific experiences dealing with arrogant, uninformed, or downright abusive physicians, and many more have been massively discouraged as they move from doctor to doctor, seeking help they cannot find. Just as rape victims feel that insensitive treatment by police and lawyers often constitutes a "second rape," so we feel that callous treatment by doctors who should know better becomes a painful "second trauma." We'll help you understand what to do when doctors get it wrong—from the well-intentioned to the inexcusably crass and unfeeling—in hopes of helping you to heal emotionally and move on.

In Chapter 3, we explain how to find a doctor who will offer you effective treatment, and how to work with such a doctor once you've found him or her. We know it's not easy to find the right doctor for sexual pain, but we'll talk you through what you need to do, every step of the way.

Finally, because your healing shouldn't have to wait until you locate the right doctor, we explain in Chapter 4 what you can do to start healing on your own. We'll talk about immediate steps you can take to feel better, both sexually and generally, and we'll help you gather your strength and hope for the healing journey ahead.

Part 2 is devoted to "Understanding the Problem." Here we talk through each one of the medical conditions that might be the source of your sexual pain. In Chapter 5, we explain the biology of pain, so you can understand exactly what's happening in your body and brain. We also explain inflammation—a medical condition that accompanies almost every form of sexual pain, and one you can begin to treat with diet, exercise, and lifestyle changes even as you seek more specific treatments. Finally, we offer a list of symptoms that will help you identify which of the other chapters in this section might apply to you.

Chapters 6 through 13 each focus on a specific medical condition that might be causing sexual pain. Each chapter discusses the biology behind the conditions, explains how your physician should be diagnosing the problems, and provides the latest information about available treatments. You'll also read stories of our patients who have battled through these conditions to find help.

In Part 3, we talk about "Overcoming the Problem," with an eye on helping you recover and move on. Chapter 14 looks specifically at how you can restore joy to your sex life—whether you are single or involved, and whether you relate sexually to men or women. In Chapter 15, we talk about how to restore trust and intimacy to sexual partnerships, friendships, and family relationships—all of which may have been affected by your ordeal. Chapter 16 helps you see how to move forward into recovery, so that your sexual healing can be complete. We also acknowledge that for some women, the process of recovery is an ongoing one—in which life can get better, but in which pain is always a potential visitor. For these women too, a joyous future awaits, even if it is sometimes shadowed by pain.

After you have completed this book, we hope you will be fortified to face the daunting task of attaining sexual health. Remember, you are not alone in your travels, and you can use this book as a medical and psychological resource and support.

We've made it our life's work to help women with pelvic pain, and we want to help you too. As you read this book, it is our deepest wish that it will give you the knowledge you need to ease your pain.

Please don't give up hope—you can get better!

AUTHORS' NOTE

The facts about and the quotes from the women interviewed are all true, but their names, ages, and occupations have been changed to protect their identities.

PART ONE

NAMING THE PROBLEM

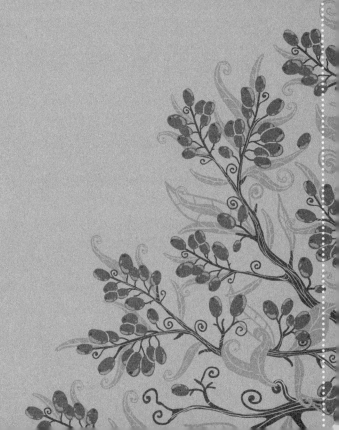

1

.....

TALKING
ABOUT
SEXUAL PAIN

I just wanted to disappear from the face of the earth. I actually thought of killing myself at times, because I felt no one understood what I was going through, and I was desperately afraid that no one could help me. I also was panicked that I could lose my job. What kept me from killing myself was an inner voice that kept telling me to keep going—to have hope. When things were really bad, I had no social life. I stopped talking to my friends, because I was tired of telling them that I wasn't feeling well.

—MELANIE, LIBRARIAN, AGE FORTY

THAT'S HOW MELANIE felt when she was coping with her sexual pain—an extremely complicated mix of symptoms and causes that took far too long for her physicians to decipher.

We are glad Melanie kept listening to her inner voice. But we are sad to think of her shutting out the voices of her friends and loved ones, because if anything can make sexual pain worse, it is the isolation of not being able to talk about it—with anyone.

SILENCE AND SEXUAL PAIN

Women who suffer from sexual pain feel isolated and confused in a way that's like no other we've ever seen.

You might confess to your coworkers that you frequently get migraines or struggle with back pain, but it's a lot harder to excuse an absence from work by saying "My clitoris was giving me a lot of trouble" or to explain the need for a special pillow on your office chair by saying "I have this awful skin condition on my vulva." Even if you have a steady partner and a great sex life, you—or your partner—may be uncomfortable talking about all the things that have gone wrong "down there," or you may feel overwhelmed by all the emotions that come up for each of you—shame, guilt, frustration, sadness, anger, isolation, confusion. If you are seeing someone new, trying to date, or living a single life, sexual pain can make you feel so alone.

You may have many reasons for not wanting to talk about sexual pain. Perhaps you feel as though you're leading a double life: There is the happy, confident persona you try to present to colleagues, neighbors, and maybe even family, friends, and partners . . . and then there is the agonized, despairing, terrified person you so often feel like in private. "No one understands what I'm going through" is a common refrain among our patients, and they are not entirely wrong. It is difficult for other people to understand how excruciating and debilitating sexual pain can be and how it can affect your core identity as a sexual, attractive woman.

"I would walk into a room and think, *Hey, I look pretty good,* and then I would feel like a farce," Stephanie admits. A banking executive at a major company for thirty years, Stephanie had spent years learning how to claim her own competence at work. Once she had achieved a sense of professional mastery, she suddenly found herself undermined by her own body when she developed sexual pain as the result of hormonal changes brought on by menopause.

"I knew I was an attractive woman, but I thought, *No one knows how miserable I feel about my body and my crotch,*" Stephanie says. "I felt really crummy about myself. My sense of self was just shattered."

For Stephanie, isolation made everything worse—but talking to people only reinforced her sense of isolation. "I shared my feelings with very few people," she explains. "I talked to my sister-in-law and a couple of other people. They felt very sad for me. I didn't get much support. They would feel mad at my husband and feel sorry for me. No one really got it."

Besides the shame, some of our patients also tell us they feel guilt. "If it weren't for my sexual and pelvic pain, my husband would have a normal wife, family, and life without so much suffering," Sandra says. A biomedical technician in her early thirties who works in a large urban hospital, Sandra is used to dealing with other people's pain, but she understandably feels defeated by her own pelvic floor dysfunction, which causes her agonizing discomfort every time she and her husband try to make love. "There are many times I feel my husband would be better off without me," she says. "Sometimes I look into his eyes and wish I could dig myself a hole and hide in it forever."

Sandra's guilt is compounded by her husband's difficulty in talking with her about their situation. "My husband is so frustrated with my continued pain," she says. "We talk sometimes, but he shuts down a lot. He deals with our situation by running. He is planning on running in the next New York City Marathon. That is how he deals with our pain." Like Stephanie, Sandra is in a double bind. She is isolated when she doesn't talk to anyone—and often feels even more isolated when she does.

Perhaps you come from a cultural or religious background where you were raised not to talk about sex. You might feel obligated to keep silent, even to the point of hiding your condition from your gynecologist. Or perhaps you were raised not to share your feelings "outside the family." If you can't trust a family member to hear your pain and help you through the hard times, you may have nowhere to go for support. Maybe you're afraid to burden your friends with endless stories of your callous doctors, your lack of energy, your insensitive partners, and your overwhelming pain.

You might also face physical challenges in meeting up with friends. Sandra, for example, walks a constant tightrope, wanting to take part in life and socialize with her friends while trying to ensure that her pain doesn't escalate or flare up. When she withdraws from the world and lives in isolation, her depression worsens, so she tries to maintain some semblance of a normal life. But sometimes, meeting with friends has a price of its own.

"The other day, I met with a friend because I was feeling so isolated. But I guess I overdid it, and that night, I was in so much pain that I wanted to scream and cry. If I do too much, my pain gets so much worse. It gets so depressing," she says. "My friendships have suffered, because my friends get tired of hearing about my pain and why I can never go out with them."

Before her problem with clitorodynia (clitoral pain), Jessie had a warm, friendly relationship with her colleagues, who were a real source of pleasure for her. She enjoyed flirting a bit with some of the men, and generally found her workmates fun to talk to. But when she began to feel sexual pain—a condition that struck just on the eve of a long business trip to India—Jessie felt cut off from the people who had once been a big part of her social life.

"I couldn't share my pain with anyone, especially since I work with all men, and I still don't tell anyone at work," says Jessie, an otherwise confident and successful business executive in her early thirties. In India, she struggled to cope as best she could. "I somehow got through my meetings and afterward would run back to my room and sit on a bag full of ice and then go down to the bar and drink. That was how I got through this horrendous trip."

From that point on, Jessie not only couldn't enjoy her life at work, but she also couldn't tell anyone what was happening to her. Suddenly, every day at work was torture—both because sitting was so painful, and because she had to work so hard to hide her discomfort.

Maybe you've had chances to talk about your sexual pain but don't want to focus on your illness. Our patient Miriam—now a healthy, vibrant woman in her early thirties—was articulate and confident in her professional life. She's earned a PhD in history, and she teaches at a prestigious academic institution and works as a policy analyst. Before developing vestibulodynia (pain in the vaginal opening), Miriam felt quite comfortable talking about her sex life, at least with her partner.

Now, Miriam says, "I am traumatized on various levels and am so angry." Part of the problem, she explains, is that she feels her illness has become her identity. "I didn't want to talk about all this—not because I was embarrassed, but because the more I talked about it, the more I was constituting an identity that I didn't want to have. I didn't want to talk about it to my friends, because I would have been creating this person who I didn't want to be. I said to myself that my sexuality and my body are intact, and this is a temporary condition. I did what I needed to do, but I didn't want to construct this mental framework. I knew if I did that, it would come back to haunt me."

Maybe you're so uncomfortable discussing sexual pain that you don't even want to bring it up to your gynecologist—even if you've made the appointment for that very reason. Many of our patients have told stories of going to the doctor, prepared to talk about their condition—and then somehow stopping short. When they returned home, they were disappointed in themselves—but they still didn't break the silence.

If you're a young woman or a teenager, you might think that a certain amount of pain is normal during sex. Maybe you've assumed that everyone finds sex painful. Or perhaps you thought the pain would go away by itself someday and then felt too embarrassed to say anything when it didn't. Many of our patients don't even tell their partners how uncomfortable they are but instead find ways to keep intercourse from lasting too long, or to avoid touch or positions that hurt. Or they simply avoid sex altogether.

Finally, if your sexual pain came on very suddenly and abruptly, as it often happens, you may simply have been in shock. You might have assumed the pain was just a fluke, or that it was caused by a yeast infection that would eventually disappear. Because sexual pain is so rarely discussed, there's a good chance you hadn't even heard of it until you developed it—which makes it even harder to bring up with a doctor or a therapist, let alone a partner, a family member, or a friend. To the pain in your body is added the pain of isolation.

THOUGHTS THAT KEEP US SILENT

- I feel like a freak.

- I don't know anyone else who's going through this.

- I can't imagine who I'd talk to about this.

- My partner doesn't understand—and he/she can't talk to anyone either.

- This can't really be happening!

- Maybe it's in my mind.

- I've never heard of this—I must be making it up.

- What if people think I'm crazy?

- Is there something wrong with me psychologically?

- Maybe I really just don't like sex.

- Maybe I really just don't like my partner or am not attracted to my partner anymore.

- I'm causing this because of my sexual hang-ups.

- I'm just not lubricating well.

- Why can't I just relax?

- I should be able to deal with this by myself.

- I'm so traumatized and embarrassed about feeling like a whole sexual part of me has been amputated that I can't talk about it.

- What if I have an STD?

➤

> - I can't afford to take care of this—I hope it just goes away.

> - I looked on the web, and they said it was all in my mind.

WHAT HAPPENS WHEN YOU DON'T TALK

Shame. Depression. Feeling like damaged goods. Self-doubt. Embarrassment. A downward spiral, in which it becomes harder and harder to reach out. Withdrawing from the relationships that once meant the most to you. Actively considering and maybe even planning suicide.

These may be the consequences of maintaining silence about your sexual pain.

We know it can be extremely difficult to find a safe way to talk about your circumstances. But the cost of keeping silent may outweigh the problem of speaking up.

Our patient Theresa is a full-time speech therapist who takes a great deal of pride and satisfaction from her busy career, and she is always concerned about presenting physical and emotional strength to others. Like many women suffering from chronic sexual and vulvar pain, Theresa always appeared completely physically and emotionally intact. The cheerful facade, however, hid quite another story.

"On a good day, my pain level was a one [on a scale from zero to ten], but on a bad day—of which I had many—my pain level went up to about a seven," Theresa says. "I would say, for the most part, I was pretty depressed and down in the dumps. I am an extremely active person, and working out is my passion. I could only work out on a very limited basis, and that added to my depression. Also, it was very hard when people who know me at the gym asked why I was taking breaks. Sometimes I had to rest during my workouts because of the pain. I usually said I had neurological pain, because it would be too uncomfortable and embarrassing to tell the truth. I always felt like I was walking around with a terrible secret."

Of course, Theresa has the right to decide how much of her condition she will disclose, and to whom. But feeling as though she had to keep a secret—one that she struggled to conceal—compounded the shame, guilt, and isolation of the disease itself. By trying always to hide her sexual pain and its symptoms, Theresa was contributing to her own sense of shame.

Theresa's dilemma intensified when her sexual pain interfered more actively with her second job as a Pilates instructor, causing her to limit the positions she was demonstrating. "One time a woman in my class asked me if I was pregnant, because I altered my teaching in the class," Theresa reports. "That was quite embarrassing."

Keeping secrets at work was bad enough, but Theresa really felt the frustration of not being able to even consider dating. "So many of my friends had boyfriends, and I couldn't even go on a date. It was just so hard," she says. "I know it's not easy when you are married or in a relationship, but at least you have a background with a man. There is no way I could explain this to a man or think about getting intimate with one."

Theresa did have a few people she could talk with, but she didn't feel she could be as open as she needed to be. "I talk to two friends about my condition and also share some feelings with my mom," she says. "But my mother worries about me all the time. My friends are very supportive, but they have no idea what to say and they have no idea what I am talking about. In the end, talking to them is a very lonely and isolating feeling."

HOW SEXUAL PAIN CAN AFFECT BODY IMAGE

Savannah, a thirty-one-year-old reproductive health worker, always thought of herself as a healthy and vibrant sexual

➤

woman—until she developed two sexual pain conditions, vestibulodynia and lichen sclerosus. Although she had a loving partner who continued to be attracted to her, her sex life was one of the first casualties of her condition.

"I'm very educated about sexual health, and that is even the business I am in," says Savannah. "I never had any sexual hang-ups and had very healthy sexual relationships until all my medical complications started. Now, my body image has totally changed. This has taken on a life of its own, and at this point in my life, I would not describe myself as a sexual person. I'm sort of closed off, and it's my own doing. I put [my sex life] off in a corner, and this is a place I never thought I would be in my life."

Although Savannah and other women do experience an altered or distorted body image, sharing feelings with other women and possibly a therapist can help women regain a healthy sense of themselves and their bodies.

BREAKING THE SILENCE

We know how difficult it can be to break the silence about sexual pain. Both of us have struggled with a variety of personal and family medical problems, and Nancy has had an ongoing battle with her own pelvic pain. We know that many people just don't understand, and that it's important to preserve a professional distance with colleagues. Family members mean well but are not always the best people to help you process your complicated feelings. We understand too that even your closest friends, relatives, and partners have their own difficult relationship to your pain. They too feel vulnerable and helpless and anxious when they consider how hard things are for you, and how little they can sometimes do to help.

We understand. But still we say, with all the depth of our personal and professional experience: Break the silence. Start talking. Find someone who will be able to know what you are going through, someone you can turn to when you're feeling low.

We realize it is overwhelming to start talking about a topic that often feels so shameful. But if you take it in baby steps, a little at a time, you will find it easier to do. Here are our suggestions for how to begin to break the silence.

Pick one person you trust to validate your feelings.
Your goal is to find someone who, when you tell them how you're feeling, is able to say, "I hear you" or "I understand." Who do you usually go to when you have a real problem? Your partner? Your friend? Your sister? Your mother?

If you genuinely feel that you can't trust anyone in your life with this topic, we urge you, in the strongest possible terms, to find an "outsider"—a therapist, religious leader, spiritual counselor, or someone else you can open up with. Even calling a hotline and speaking anonymously over the phone is better than not opening up to anyone. Humans are social animals; we aren't meant to be isolated. Intense pain can send you scurrying for safety, away from the rest of the world. But then you will face the added pain of being disconnected from others.

Talk to your partner, but find someone else too.
If you're in an ongoing sexual relationship, we urge you to talk about what's happening with your partner. In many relationships, sex is our affirmation of closeness. If you temporarily lose the ability to be sexual together and you're also not talking about this major issue for the two of you, you're driving a wedge into the heart of your relationship. You don't necessarily have to have extensive, blow-by-blow discussions with your partner, but don't shut him or her out. Keep open a space where the two of you can be in this together, not apart.

Having said that, we also think it's very important to have someone to talk to who is *not* your partner—whether friend, relative, or therapist. There will be times when your partner is overwhelmed with his or her own feelings about your situation and won't have the emotional space to support you as you would like. And there will be times when you need to blow off steam *about* your partner, not *to* your partner. You might also feel that it's easier for someone you're not sexually intimate with to hear the most extreme and uncensored versions of your fears, frustration, anger, and hopelessness, while with your partner you strive to present a more balanced picture. Also, if your partner is a man, you might just want a woman to talk to—someone who understands in a different way how it feels to be in your situation.

Be selective, and be willing to stop talking to someone who's not supportive.
You're looking for someone who will validate your feelings, not minimize them. If the person you're speaking with says, "Oh, you'll get over it" or "Try not to worry," find someone else. If you can see that the person you're speaking with is overwhelmed with worry for you, worry for herself, or general discomfort, change the subject and look for someone else.

It can be difficult to search for a support person when you're already feeling anxious or defeated, but we urge you to find the resources in yourself to keep looking. Although we have a lot of faith that you can find the treatment you need and significantly improve your condition, you're most likely in for a long, difficult journey. Breaking the silence and finding someone to "be in it with you" is a significant part of what will enable you to keep going.

Try to normalize the topic for yourself.
Many of us talk with our friends about PMS, cramps, childbirth, nursing problems, hot flashes, and other "female conditions." We also talk about other medical conditions, such as diabetes and cancer. Although sexual pain is unique in many ways, it also has similarities to other female issues and to other illnesses. When you are looking for a friend or loved one to talk with, see if you can put this problem in the same category as those others.

Fight the feeling that you are "defective."

If there's one idea that comes up with virtually all of our sexual-pain patients, it's that one. Every woman with a sexual-pain condition has to fight the feeling that there is something wrong with her, and this sense of being defective is part of what keeps so many silent.

It can be difficult to fight this feeling, we know. But remember: As many as one woman in five is going through some version of what you are going through. You might even discover that the person you speak to has had her own history of sexual pain that she was unwilling to speak about. Almost certainly she has something she is ashamed of or anxious about, something she fears makes her defective or incomplete. In talking about your own fears and shame, you may find yourself helping her as well as yourself.

Keep your eyes on the prize—and be realistic.

If you visualize how good it will feel to not be alone with your pain, that may give you the courage and stamina to keep looking for a support system. At the same time, virtually every woman we've spoken with who has a support system is aware both of its strengths and of its weaknesses.

WOMEN WHO HAVE BROKEN THE SILENCE

Savannah, the reproductive health worker mentioned earlier in this chapter, has built herself an extraordinary network of support. "My support system is my partner, my best friend, my therapist, and my closest friends," she says. "My therapist really gets it. And I am able to talk about the nitty-gritty details with my best friend. This helps a lot."

But even Savannah feels isolated sometimes. "I go through my periods of feeling shitty and sorry for myself, but things have never gotten that bad that I have wanted to end my life," she says. "However, all my medical issues can be overwhelming at times, and there are times I hit rock bottom and feel hopeless. I do allow myself to fall apart sometimes, but I don't want to stay in that place. For me, it's better when I come out of a hard time and hit it head on. . . . None of my closest friends are dealing with these issues, and that is hard. When I was attending a yoga class, I met another woman who also had vulvovaginal issues. It was a mind-blowing experience to talk with someone else who is going through the same thing. It can be so isolating otherwise."

Likewise, Lucy—a twenty-seven-year-old editor at a fashion magazine—relies on a support system but acknowledges its limits. "I am lucky because my sister lives in my building, and I tell her everything, and she is a tremendous support," she says. "My mom knows basically what is going on but I don't tell her I can't have sex. I only tell her that I can't use a tampon, but I assume she knows the real story. What I tell my friends is that the Pill screwed up my body, but I don't feel comfortable sharing anything else with them. I don't want them to know that Dave and I aren't having sex. I would just find that way too embarrassing."

Karen—a woman in her late twenties who works in the fashion industry—also treasures her support system while acknowledging its limits. "After my husband, I would have to say my mom is my biggest support," she says. "I can tell her everything. I also talk to a couple of friends who have been very understanding. But I feel if I talk too much, I will turn my friends off. I know in the back of my mind that even though they are supportive, they don't totally understand what I am going through. And I don't want to be a downer."

Although Karen feels generally supported by her friends, she's selective about what she says to whom. "I have a very close friend, and I discuss everything with her. We are never embarrassed to discuss sexual issues. But I don't discuss this with my mother-in-law in depth. She knows just the tip of the iceberg. She knows that I have a bladder condition but she doesn't know about my vulvovaginal problems. Only a very few select people know the ins and outs of every day."

Karen also found herself being selective about what she told her colleagues. "My friend and former manager know the most about my condition," she says. "But otherwise I find it very difficult to deal with at work.

The hardest thing is when we have office parties, people bring in special food that they know will not aggravate my condition. I really appreciate what people do for me but wish they would stop bringing things in for me. What was very difficult is when I got transferred to another department, and I had a new manager, and I had to tell her the details of my painful bladder syndrome. She is pretty good, because she gets urinary tract infections. I had to tell her, because of all my doctor appointments."

Although Karen would have preferred not sharing her medical details at work, she ultimately found a way to be at peace with it. "I read on [an online support network] that people are embarrassed to tell people at work when they have to go to the bathroom," she says. "I just do what I have to do. I usually say I have a bladder condition and don't go into details."

DEPRESSION AND HOPELESSNESS

Anyone who suffers from chronic pain must cope with depression, and at times, even a sense of hopelessness and despair. Living with pain is exhausting, and sometimes it feels as though it just sucks every bit of life out of you. There are times when getting out of bed in the morning is more than you can bear. And sometimes you may feel completely hopeless that there will ever be a reduction in your pain level.

All of these are normal reactions to living with pain. Sometimes giving in to your depression is a healthy coping mechanism. Of course, if your depression becomes debilitating, it's time to seek counseling. It's also important to reach out to someone in your support system when your emotional pain becomes unbearable. But if you have days when all you can do is lie in bed and watch mindless TV, that is okay. In fact, giving yourself permission to fall apart at times and become nonfunctioning is a healthy coping mechanism, as long as it doesn't last too long.

WHEN DEPRESSION GOES TOO FAR

Depression is part of any pain condition. You cannot escape it. But your depression shouldn't consume you. If you notice any of the following signs of severe clinical depression, talk with your doctor or therapist:

- a loss of appetite;

- a change in sleep patterns, such as inability to fall asleep, waking up in the middle of the night, or sleeping most of the day;

- spending a week or more in bed;

- spending hours at a time crying or sitting numbly;

- finding yourself unable to enjoy any of the activities or treats that used to lift your spirits;

- withdrawing from close relationships and actively driving people away;

- not going to work; and/or

- creating a specific plan for suicide, such as overdosing on pills or slitting your wrists.

FREQUENT THOUGHTS OF SUICIDE

When you live with chronic pain, it is perfectly normal at times to think that ending your life would be better than living with unending pain. In fact, knowing that you have the choice to kill yourself can be an important aspect of feeling in control of your life at a time when chronic pain threatens to disempower you completely.

However, if you think so specifically of suicide that you actually begin to work on a plan, then your thoughts have become dangerous. Simply thinking about suicide or even imagining a plan is not dangerous—in fact, most of the women we interviewed for this book have done so. Some women even told us that they would rather be hit by a bus than live with their pain. But if you find yourself beginning to work out the details—where you would buy the pills, or what time of day you would arrange to slit your wrists—then you need to share your thoughts with a loved one or a therapist.

IF YOU HAVE THOUGHTS OF SUICIDE

- Remind yourself that it is normal, and you are not crazy—you are simply asserting control over your life.

- Think about the times you did not feel such intense pain, and remind yourself that this degree of pain is only temporary—there will be medications or treatment to help minimize your pain, and there will be times you feel better.

- Remember that you don't actually want to die—just to end your pain. Even though you have reasons to want to end your life, you also have reasons to live. Ask yourself to find one or more reasons.

- Create mental images to remind yourself which parts of life you would miss if you were no longer here. Images such as loving times with your family, snuggling with your child or partner, or completing work that is important to you can help you hold on.

Ongoing Stress in Your Relationships

Communicating with your loved ones is vital to reducing the stress in your relationships. But no matter how hard you try, there will be times when you feel so cranky and exhausted from your pain that normal conversation with your partner or a friend may be too difficult. Accept that this will be a challenge, and ask your loved ones to accept it also. You will all have an easier time if you acknowledge that some days you will have to leave each other alone. Just make sure to maintain some degree of connection on the days when it's possible.

Letting your partner know how you feel is important, and asking your partner how he or she feels is equally important. You don't have to protect each other from your feelings; in fact, trying to do so usually results in frustration and anger.

One of our patients, Lynn, tells her friends how she feels and asks them to accommodate her. "When I am having a bad day and I have plans with my friends, they try to adapt our plans so I can participate," she says. "It was hard for me to let them do that, but I've learned that it's important for all of us. This way, the relationships can continue. I've learned not to be so proud, and they are relieved that there is something they can do for me."

WHEN THE PAIN IS OVERWHELMING

- Use a 1-to-10 pain scale to let your partner or support person know how you are feeling.

- Tell your partner or support person what you need, both physically and emotionally, when you are having a difficult time. Don't be a stoic—that usually backfires.

➤

➤
- Recognize your loved ones' feelings, and tell them that you understand how difficult this is for all of you.

- Encourage communication, and tell your loved ones not to protect you by hiding their feelings.

FINDING YOUR OWN WAY

Having to cope with sexual pain can be a profoundly disempowering experience. A core portion of your identity has seemingly been taken from you, often suddenly, and with no explanation. As you work to reclaim your female and sexual identity, you want as much as possible to assert your control over the things you can control—and that includes how, when, and with whom you share your feelings about your condition.

We support your right to make your own decisions about how to reach out for the support you need—but we urge you to reach out, and to keep reaching out. Sometimes a person who was good to talk to suddenly "drops out" or becomes less satisfying; sometimes a person you never thought you could trust appears to you in a different light.

Like anything else, building and relying on a support system is a process, and the key to making it work is putting in continuous efforts to sustain this support. Despite all the challenges that may arise, creating a support system for yourself is one of the best things you can possibly do while coping with sexual pain.

2

.....

DOCTORS
WHO GET IT
WRONG

*The first doctor I went to was horrible. All he did was talk to me—
he didn't even really examine me—and that's how he came up with
his diagnosis! Then he gave me a medication that made me worse.
I was in excruciating pain, and I couldn't get another appointment
with him for six months. I cried every night. . . . I just don't trust
any doctor anymore. I feel I have posttraumatic stress disorder
from going to so many doctors who treated me so poorly.*

—Karen, a fashion designer in her late twenties

*After visiting seven doctors, I finally went back to my gynecolo-
gist, who told me that all my symptoms were in my head. He said
I should be getting better with the creams. And when I asked him
how he could explain the itching in my vulva, and told him it had
gotten to the point where I could barely walk, he told me I needed
psychological help.*

—Mary, a teacher in her forties

T HESE ARE JUST two stories of women who had bad experiences with
doctors. Believe us when we tell you we could easily have supplied you
with a hundred more. Most of our sexual-pain patients have seen at least
half a dozen physicians before they come to us. When coping with the agony
and despair of sexual pain, dealing with doctors can be one of the worst
aspects.

ENDURING MEDICAL TRAUMA

Many women report having been misdiagnosed, given inappropriate medications, treated insensitively, or told their pain was psychosomatic. And based
on our experience, when doctors realize they're unable to provide effective
treatment, it's very rare they can even refer the patient to someone who can.

Some women with incorrect diagnoses have even undergone unnecessary surgeries (such as hysterectomies) that actually increased their sexual
pain or worsened their conditions.

Most doctors and gynecologists are capable healthcare practitioners
who are equipped to deal with other complex gynecological conditions.
However, for a variety of reasons, most physicians are surprisingly ignorant
when it comes to sexual pain. Many are not comfortable with this area of
medicine and therefore avoid educating themselves.

The degree of incompetence, insensitivity, and indifference among
gynecologists, other specialists, and general practitioners is hard to over-
state. Deborah is frequently shocked by how little awareness even the most
enlightened MDs have of sexual pain, and how unwilling they are to learn
about it. As we'll see later in this chapter, treating sexual pain often requires
more time, care, and knowledge than other conditions. Doctors under pressure to move through a long day's worth of fifteen-minute appointments are
unlikely to devote one or two hours to take a full history of a sexual-pain
patient, or to work through the various possibilities for her diagnosis and
cure. Doctors who are uncomfortable talking about sex—and all too many
are—will not want to engage with the problems of sexual pain. And doctors

who like believing they are equipped to deal with any illness or injury will not be happy to encounter a condition they don't immediately know how to treat. As a result, women asking doctors for help with their sexual pain are likely to meet with polite indifference at best, arrogant insensitivity at worst.

If you are suffering from sexual pain, it may have taken every ounce of your courage to make an appointment with your doctor and to then reveal intimate details of your life. To then encounter offensive statements can feel like a terrible emotional assault.

As a result, by the time women reach our offices, many seem like survivors of a natural disaster. Many feel abandoned, betrayed, or abased by the medical system. Although they know there is something physically wrong, many women start believing the comments they have heard, or may blame themselves for their pain. Having lost all faith in doctors, they now feel bereft—for if the medical system can't offer them effective treatment and relief from pain, who can?

DOCTOR QUOTES: THE WORST OF THE WORST

If you finally mustered the courage to see your doctor about your sexual pain, and he or she made what seemed like outlandish and ignorant comments, you are not alone. Statements like the following are unfortunately common.

- "Have a glass of wine."

- "Maybe you should see a therapist."

- "It's all in your head."

- "You are catastrophizing your pain."

- "You just need to relax."

➤

> - "Your attitude is making things worse."

- "Just grin and bear it."

- "I don't see anything wrong."

- "There is nothing physically wrong with you."

- "There is nothing more I can do for you."

- "There must be something wrong in your relationship."

- "Get over it."

- "You are better."

- And unbelievable but true: "Tell your boyfriend he'd better get a new girlfriend."

THE AFTEREFFECTS OF MEDICAL MISTREATMENT

The experience of being mistreated by one doctor after another leaves its mark on women suffering from sexual pain. If you've been to multiple doctors for your condition, you might well be struggling with one of the following psychological effects:

Self-Blame

Perhaps, like our patient Melanie, you have come to blame yourself for not getting better, as though you were somehow at fault instead of the doctors who couldn't cure you. "I couldn't stand to think it was the doctors failing me, because then, who was going to help me?" she tells us. "I had to believe I was the one who hadn't done enough to make myself well again. I still don't know what else I could have done—but it was almost like I was afraid to believe it was them instead of me."

We can understand why women start to blame themselves. First, many people tend to defer to authority, to assume that if a relationship with an authority figure is not working, they themselves must be at fault. Second, given that women with sexual pain are dependent upon doctors to cure them, the idea that a doctor might not be able to help—that he or she might not even be competent to treat you—is very frightening indeed. Better to believe that you are the problem and leave the doctors to their godlike authority.

Self-Doubt

Our patient Mary, a part-time teacher in her forties, was incorrectly diagnosed and therefore incorrectly treated for her skin condition. When her symptoms came back, she called the doctor who diagnosed her, but he had no idea why she was once again symptomatic. He told her that the medicine he'd given her should have worked, and that maybe she should consider getting some emotional help, because at this point, her condition might be psychologically rooted.

Mary's initial response was anger. "I thought this doctor was arrogant when I first met him," she says. "But then, when he told me the itching was in my head, I almost put my fist through the phone and ripped his head off. I told him there is no way this could be in my head, and that he was one of the most unsympathetic and arrogant doctors I had ever been to. He told me that he never heard this complaint from other patients, and that my response was even more evidence of a psychological problem."

At first, Mary remained angry. But then she began to wonder if the doctor was right. "When no one can help you, and everyone insists that your problem doesn't exist, it's very hard to stay with what you know to be true," she says. Of all the upsetting things that happened to her in the course of her illness, she considers one of the worst to be the way she allowed the doctor to "get inside her head" and cause her to doubt her own perceptions. "Feeling like I was crazy—or at least wondering whether I was—that was a nightmare," she says.

Likewise, Miriam—the history professor we met in Chapter 1—began to doubt herself when one doctor after another told her that her problem was psychological.

"I do want my life back, but in some way, the illness has become a friend," Miriam says. "It's like a cigarette—you know it's killing you and that it is bad for you, but it becomes your companion, and it is very hard to give up. So if any doctor told me I was crazy, I started to believe them, because I wondered if I was using this as a crutch."

Desensitization

It's hard going through one gynecological exam after another, even for women who are comfortable with their bodies and their nakedness. Theresa—the speech therapist we met in Chapter 1—says that she has always been comfortable with her sexuality. But the multiple exams she underwent left their mark.

"I've had to get used to being examined in that private part of my body," Theresa says. "I see my gynecologist once a month when I should be seeing her once a year. I've had to desensitize myself, so I now feel like when someone is examining my genitals, they could be looking at my elbow or knee. You have to do this to tolerate such an invasion of a body part that shouldn't be looked at so often."

Likewise, Miriam feels that the trauma of her treatments continues to affect her. Although she considers herself cured of her sexual pain, she does not consider herself cured psychologically.

"I still have difficulties. I have never been a person who I consider to be inhibited, but I've always been a person who is rather private. I've always handled my private life privately. I was never the girl to kiss and tell. So this sexual pain pushed me to be a lot more open about my sexuality and my partnership, and to be way out of my comfort zone. And the feeling that I got was that my sexuality and private parts were on display, because I had so many people examining and discussing them. There is this whole medicalization of my sexuality—there is this constant reporting about my sexuality and whether I have intercourse or not. It just took everything away from me. I have a huge problem with my libido now. I would say that my whole sex life is deranged right now. I think what will help me is to stop interacting with medical professionals," she says.

And Miriam's coping mechanism for this invasion turned into a problem of its own. "It's almost as if I developed a stage persona . . . to help me talk about things that are nobody's business. I feel like this is something I only want to share with my partner—this belongs only to him and me and not to the public. And now I have the problem of how to get rid of this stage persona."

WHERE DO THEY GO WRONG?

"Insensitive." "Arrogant." "Incompetent." "Uncaring."

Surely these are not terms doctors want to hear in reference to themselves. So why do so many patients report these things? Of course, some doctors simply *are* insensitive, arrogant, and/or incompetent. You could also argue that in a field where many of the practitioners are still men and all of the patients are women, traditional male–female power relations enter into the picture.

But many otherwise capable and compassionate doctors—including women—consistently fail the women who come to them for help with sexual pain. Why?

In our view, there are a few key reasons:

The Lack of Information

To a shocking extent, doctors simply don't know about sexual pain: how it starts, how it worsens, how to treat it. Deborah is often surprised, when examining a woman who is clearly suffering from a particular condition, to learn that the previous physician misdiagnosed her or offered no diagnosis at all. Clearly, many doctors simply don't know what to look for or how to interpret their findings.

Some of this has to do with the nature of the ob-gyn specialty. People who go into obstetrics are primarily interested in supporting women through pregnancy and delivering babies. People who go into gynecology are focused on surgery, hormonal problems, menstrual disorders, contraception, menopause, and well-woman care. If gynecologists specialize further, it may be in cancer or infertility—better-known and more easily talked-about fields. There's no focus on sexual pain in medical education, no residency rotation, no fellowships. The only reason Deborah ended up with the level of education she has in the field is that she became interested in it and pursued it on her own. Most doctors see no reason to do that.

The Focus of Western Medicine

Education about sexual pain is lacking in most medical schools—in fact, there's little education about chronic pain of any kind. Western medicine is generally focused on acute problems—dramatic illnesses or surgeries for which there is a clear-cut treatment and cure. Chronic illness is poorly understood, and virtually nothing in our medical system—how doctors are educated, how practices are run, how insurance companies reimburse doctors—is set up to deal with it.

Of course, some cutting-edge research is being done on the treatment and management of chronic pain. But for the most part, Western medicine is good at relieving acute pain and treating acute illnesses, not at getting at the underlying causes of chronic pain or managing long-term, ongoing conditions.

The Need to "Know It All"

Whether or not doctors expect themselves to be all-knowing, patients often do expect that of their physicians. And most doctors feel very uncomfortable admitting they don't know something. Many physicians apparently prefer to offer an incorrect diagnosis than to not give one at all, which would disappoint the patients and themselves. It can sometimes seem as though doctors are given a medical magic hat upon graduation from medical school, and when they're faced with an unknown condition, their instruction manual tells them to dip into the hat and pull out a diagnosis—any diagnosis. These arbitrary pronouncements seem to give many physicians a sense of power and control when they in fact feel the least empowered and secure.

Kate was a successful film producer. She has spent the past seventeen years trying to undo damage from a minor surgical procedure she had in the early 1980s. "A couple of months after this procedure, I developed searing pain around the site," she says. "And then something very odd happened: The entire left side of my body, from my head to my ankle, developed horrendous pain. And the vulvovaginal pain was petrifying. I went to the gynecologist who did the procedure, and he said, in utter sincerity, 'You know, there are other ways to have sex.' I almost fainted when he said this, because he was a top doctor in the area," says Kate.

"My feeling about doctors is that they don't like not knowing what is wrong with you, because if they don't know, there is something wrong with *them*. So they immediately flip it and put it on you. You can almost see it in their faces—you see when they don't have the answers. My doctor didn't even acknowledge that I was having pain. I was incensed."

The Problem of the "Difficult Patient"

Let's look at things from the doctor's point of view for a moment. You're a doctor. You're busy, stressed, and overwhelmed with a huge load of patients, all of whom are expecting you to fix whatever ails them—as quickly and cheaply as possible. When you give them diets and lifestyle changes, they don't comply. When you give them a course of pills to take, they may still not comply. When they're giving you information about their problem, they don't know the difference between key facts needed to make an accurate diagnosis and extraneous details that take time away from other patients who need you more. Your patients are sick, scared, and worried about the future—but your day is blocked into fifteen-minute appointments, and you're already running late. You really don't have time to deal with their emotions. Besides, if you bonded emotionally with every patient you saw every day, you'd be a burnt-out wreck. You have to keep some professional distance.

Some doctors are an extreme example of this model, and some—like Deborah—are at the other end of the spectrum. But every physician struggles with the problem of too little time and too many emotional demands from ailing and anxious patients. In this context, there is a certain kind of patient doctors frequently refer to as "difficult." Whatever the doctor does for them, they're never satisfied. However the doctor treats them, it doesn't work. They're always back with more complaints, more emotion, more pain. Doctors are only human. When given the choice between a patient whose problems never seem to go away and one whose pain can be relieved in a single visit, who do you think they'd prefer to deal with?

Of course, the word "difficult" has two meanings here. There is the difficult case—the illness that is hard to treat, the pain that is almost impossible to relieve. Virtually all sexual-pain patients fall into that category. Then there is the difficult personality—the person who is never satisfied, the hypochondriac who is never cured. Many doctors confuse the two, treating women with sexual pain as though it were somehow their fault that their stubborn, intractable conditions refuse to respond to the doctor's well-meaning treatment. This problem is compounded because many doctors—male and female—tend in any case to see women patients as complainers.

We're not excusing this kind of response. Doctors take an oath to help people, and if they don't want to deal with sick people and their emotions, they shouldn't go into medicine. But the dynamic of the "difficult patient" is part of the reason so many women with sexual pain go from doctor to doctor to doctor, frantically seeking a physician who won't see them as difficult, but instead as someone who desperately needs their help.

The Structure of U.S. Healthcare
We've just looked at the problem from a psychological point of view. Now let's look at the economics. In the United States, most doctors get paid based on how many patients they see—that's just a fact of the healthcare system.

They cut up their day into fifteen-minute increments because, given the realities of insurance and Medicare and HMOs, that's the only way they can pay for their offices and salaries and malpractice insurance policies.

In this context, many doctors are simply not willing to deal with a patient who requires more than that fifteen-minute visit. They don't have time to take the long, complicated medical histories that, as you'll see in Part 2, are often critical to establishing a diagnosis. They don't have time to do the research that might lead them to discover new and promising treatments for a type of illness they don't understand and will need to learn about. Even if they wanted to, they don't have time to cope with the emotional needs of a woman in sexual pain.

Let's say a doctor realizes that a sexual-pain patient will take six times the attention of another type of gynecological patient. (Based on Deborah's experience, six times is probably an underestimate.) Do we really expect that doctor to voluntarily reduce his or her income to that extent, especially when he or she is still struggling to pay off the bills from medical school and is looking at how to pay for her kids' college tuition? Even if you could show this hypothetical doctor that taking on a sexual-pain patient *is* affordable, in the doctor's mind, that patient is a drain on an already limited source of time, money, and energy.

Deborah, who insists on gearing her treatment toward the patient's needs, has had to stop accepting insurance. The only way she can afford to run her practice is to see each woman for as long as it takes to explore the problem—and then to charge accordingly. She simply can't fit a comprehensive, in-depth style of care into the cookie-cutter segments that virtually every healthcare organization demands. Here's Deborah, describing her own experience organizing a practice focusing on sexual-pain patients.

When I first began to practice as a gynecologist, I had to see patients every fifteen minutes. We offered the full range of ob-gyn treatment, and of course we had a lot of pregnant women coming in, as well as a high volume of patients generally. In that context, it's just not possible to spend much time with each patient. Because we were taking insurance, we were limited in how much we could charge per visit, and so basically, economics forced us to restrict how long a patient visit could be.

As it happened, we added several midwives to that practice, and they began to concentrate on the obstetrics patients, so that gradually, I was able to take over more of the gynecological patients. Eventually I realized that patients with gynecological problems—especially sexual pain—simply needed more time. They had to be booked differently, and I began to do that.

I came to realize that I had to make a choice: I could treat women with serious gynecological problems, or I could be involved in helping women through pregnancy and delivery. But I felt I really couldn't do both effectively.

My partner (Dena Harris, MD) and I decided to open another, smaller, gynecology-only practice, and there, gradually, we began not accepting insurance. I wasn't happy about the choice, but I realized it was the best option available. If insurance would reimburse us only, say, $60 per patient visit—based on their estimate of what a fifteen-minute visit was worth—we simply couldn't cover our overhead and accept that payment for a woman who needed ninety minutes or two hours to explain a complicated history, so that we could really get to the bottom of her condition. If we'd continued taking insurance, we would have gone bankrupt!

Now we give every patient the time she needs—and we charge accordingly. It's not a perfect solution by any means, but it does allow us to give in-depth, extensive treatment to complicated conditions, including sexual pain.

We've shared this personal look at Deborah's practice because we want you to be able to look at your own doctor through that lens. If the doctor you're seeing doesn't accept insurance, you may well be given a longer first-time visit—and a bigger bill. If your doctor does accept insurance, you may ultimately have to convince the doctor to get creative, because it's very unlikely that he or she will be able to treat you or even to diagnose you in a fifteen-minute visit. (See the boxed text "Creative Ways to Work with Doctors Who Accept Insurance" in Chapter 3.)

Again, this structural problem is no excuse for treating women arrogantly or callously, let alone for giving incorrect diagnoses or inadequate treatment. If doctors aren't equipped to handle complicated cases of sexual pain, they need to find physicians who are, and to refer their patients to those doctors. Though we're not pardoning mistreatment, it's important to acknowledge that the difficulty of finding a physician who has the resources to help sexual-pain patients is at least in part a structural problem.

The Fragmented Approach to Care

One of the biggest challenges in treating sexual-pain patients is how often the usual approach doesn't work. Most doctors are used to relying on diagnostic tests—for example, pap smears, biopsies—and other tools that give a straight answer about what the problem is. Many cases of sexual pain are caused by nerve pain, and there are few tests for that.

Most gynecologists are used to treating specific medical conditions—an irregular menstrual flow, a lump, a pregnancy. They're not necessarily comfortable with discussions of sex, let alone with giving sexual advice for positions or approaches to sex that might make it easier to cope with sexual pain. Sexual medicine is still considered part of psychiatry, not gynecology, and so women with sexual pain can't get holistic treatment for any associated desire, arousal, or orgasmic problems in one place. Many women do not realize that to see a "sex therapist" for help with sexual functioning, they must enter the realm of psychiatrically trained MDs and psychologists for care, since gynecologists receive the bare minimum of formal training in sexual dysfunction and most do not have expertise to counsel or treat in this area.

Finally, most doctors are used to working solo. But sexual pain is complex and draws upon many different specialties: orthopedics, urology, dermatology, gastroenterology, and neurology, as well as physiatry, physical therapy, and counseling. Medicine isn't usually set up for a team approach—yet that's what sexual-pain patients need.

Most physicians aren't even oriented toward giving referrals. It would be wonderful, for example, if gynecologists who didn't want to deal with sexual pain at least made it their business to find one or two specialists in their geographic area who were able to treat it, and then to refer their sexual-pain patients to those specialists. But, as we've seen, most physicians expect themselves to know everything. It's hard for them to admit they don't know something, to call upon a team, and to make referrals. Even when referrals are finally made, women may receive disconnected care—one specialist advising one treatment, and another pushing his own treatment from his own field, with no discussion or consensus or workable system to coordinate the care of the patient. The medical and economic systems that doctors work in discourage connected, smooth collaboration, leaving the average patient confused and anxious.

KNOWLEDGE IS POWER

Once again, we're in no way trying to excuse doctors who leave patients traumatized by their arrogance, cluelessness, insensitivity, and incompetence. We are sharing this perspective for two reasons.

First, we don't want you to take the bad treatment personally. When you're entering the medical system, you're entering a whole culture that's not set up to help people with sexual pain. If a doctor can't talk about sex, that is his or her own hang-up; it's not your fault. If a doctor suggests a treatment that doesn't work, then that was the wrong treatment; again, not your fault. If a doctor has no clue what the problem is, then that's because of his or her medical ignorance; once again, not your fault.

Second, we know that informed doctors and patients can work together to change the way the system works. There are many ways in which the care for patients with complicated problems is getting better. Knowledge is being shared among the many different specialties and professional societies engaged in our field, a result of programs created by the International Pelvic Pain Society, the International Society for the Study of Vulvovaginal Disease, and the International Society for the Study of Women's Sexual Health. In addition, close collaboration between patients and professionals in the National Vulvodynia Association (NVA) is advancing knowledge in many ways: funding research, advocating for government support, and joining with other groups to educate and to advance new diagnosis and treatment options for chronic sexual pain.

We have great optimism that those of us working to improve the system by educating our colleagues will be successful.

IF A DOCTOR HAS TREATED YOU BADLY

- Tell the doctor.

- Write the doctor a letter.

- Write a letter to the health center or hospital administrator.

- Find another woman seeing the same doctor and vent—you might find it therapeutic.

- Go online and post about the doctor.

- Try to find other patients and take group action.

- Report them to your state medical board and to their professional association.

3
·····

HELPING
YOUR DOCTOR
GET IT RIGHT

Before the diagnosis, I thought I was totally nuts, and I felt like a
sexual freak. When I finally received the correct diagnosis, I at least
felt like I wasn't going crazy!

—CLAIRE, A FORMER FUTURES TRADER IN HER MIDFORTIES

THERE IS BOTH good news and bad news to share with you in this chapter. The good news is that there *is* good medical care out there for you. You will be able to find a doctor who can offer you effective, appropriate treatment, and who will treat you with respect.

The bad news is that you may need to visit several doctors before you find the person who is right for you. The medical field is full of physicians who aren't educated about sexual pain, who don't want "difficult" clients taking up too much of their time, or who are simply not willing to listen to their patients and treat them with respect. So you might have to go through quite a few MDs before you find the one who will give you the treatment you need. You may also need to find some creative ways to work with the physicians that you do find—and this chapter will help you with that.

We wish you could find the right doctor with a single phone call, but the sad truth is that you may have to devote a significant amount of time seeking a physician who can truly help you. Sensitive, caring, and open-minded doctors can be found, but you'll need diligence and perseverance to identify a sexual-pain expert you can trust—either a good gynecologist or a women's health nurse-practitioner.

We'll give you the information and resources you need to either find a specialist or to "make" one, by passing on what you have learned to a doctor who is willing to learn. What you'll have to provide for yourself is the courage and determination to keep going through what may well be a long and arduous search. We wish that weren't the situation—but it probably is. Please, do whatever you can to get the support you need, because finding or "making" a good doctor is crucial to your recovery—and you're worth it.

Here's one more piece of good news: Our book will help you every step of the way. So whatever you do, don't give up. You deserve good care—and you can find it. We promise.

STEP ONE: DECIDE WHAT YOU WANT IN A DOCTOR

If you live in a large urban area or near hospitals, clinics, or universities that feature a selection of gynecological specialists, you may be lucky enough to have a few candidates to interview. If this is so, it's important to know in advance what you're looking for in a doctor, so that you'll know when you've found the right one.

But even if your choices are more limited, we still encourage you to clarify the attributes that are most important to you. Knowing what you care about most will help you decide when a particular MD feels like a good compromise as opposed to a bad one.

Here are some potential attributes that you might value in an MD. Just for insight into your own priorities, rate them in order of importance from 1 to 7—1 being the most important to you and 7 being the least important.

___ knowledgeable

___ open-minded

___ able to engage in a partnership with a patient

___ accessible, not too busy

___ empathetic, caring

___ good bedside manner

___ easily reachable online through a website or through email

As you consider these qualities, please remember: Whether or not you care about a physician's bedside manner, you should never tolerate a doctor who is dismissive of your ideas and feelings. For example, if a doctor says, "Don't worry, I don't need your help. I know what is wrong with you, and I can definitely fix you," you should probably be a little suspicious. That kind of arrogance usually precludes "out of the box" thinking—and "out of the box" thinking is almost certainly what will be needed to cure sexual pain, particularly if you've been suffering longer than six months.

Of course, a kind, caring, and warm doctor is the most desirable. But you can't always find a physician like this. If a doctor is not the warm and fuzzy type but is willing to listen to some of your ideas and then follow up with a little research, that might be enough.

STEP TWO: USE YOUR RESOURCES

Ideally, you'll find a caring, sensitive doctor who is already educated in sexual pain. But that may not be possible, especially if you don't live in a large urban area. You may have to settle for a sexual-pain specialist who may not have the most sensitive bedside manner, or who otherwise isn't ideal for you. Don't settle for anyone who doesn't treat you with respect, however. That is a bottom-line, nonnegotiable requirement.

If you can't find a specialist you trust—or if you can't find one at all— your next step is to seek someone who is not educated about sexual pain but who is willing to learn, a gynecologist, a family practitioner, an internist, or a nurse-practitioner with a focus on women's healthcare. (Later in this chapter we'll show you how to help an open-minded physician learn about treating sexual pain.)

Your first step is to gather names of some doctors who are close enough to visit. Here's our breakdown of how to conduct your search:

Contact organizations that help women with sexual pain.

To find a doctor in your area who's interested in sexual pain, you can refer to lists put out by the following organizations: the International Pelvic Pain Society (IPPS), the International Society for the Study of Vulvovaginal Disease (ISSVD), and the International Society for the Study of Women's Sexual Health (ISSWSH). You should also join the National Vulvodynia Association (NVA), a helpful support organization that has a list of MDs, and that will keep you updated on the research and treatments for vulvar pain and all types of painful sex. We also highly recommend the NVA's on-line patient learning program. (For URLs and other contact information, see the Resources section, at the back of the book.)

Work your way through regular gynecologists.

If the above organizations' lists don't show any doctor in your area, your next step is to find a gynecologist who is interested in sexual pain already or who is willing to become educated on the topic. The American College of Obstetrics and Gynecology (ACOG) can help you find board-certified gynecologists who are close enough for you to visit.

Use word of mouth.

Call a local hospital's women's clinic or labor and delivery unit, and find an experienced nurse to talk to. Nurses tend to know who the good doctors are and which doctors are open to learning more.

Also ask local general practitioners, physical therapists, psychotherapists, psychiatrists, and sexologists if they know of a doctor who's educated about sexual pain or one who's sensitive, caring, and open to learning.

You may also want to ask friends and trusted colleagues how they feel about their gynecologists; you may get a great recommendation that way.

Once you have a few names, check them out on your state medical board website (see the Resources section). You probably won't find much detail, but you can at least assure yourself that there are no pending charges or complaints against the doctors you're considering.

BEWARE OF MEDICAL ARROGANCE

In some specialties, such as surgery, arrogance may not matter in a physician—it might even be a good thing, allowing him or her to work confidently under difficult circumstances. But in a field such as sexual pain—where cases are often so complex, and where your feelings are an important part of the mix—an arrogant physician is far less likely to be a good fit for you. Doctors who think they know everything and who are not open to other opinions may not have the kind of creativity you will need down the road, let alone the kind of sensitivity.

STEP THREE: PREPARE FOR YOUR APPOINTMENT

There are ten things you should do in preparation for your first appointment with a new doctor.

Collect and organize your medical documents.

Gather all your previous records and tests, and make copies for the doctor to keep and review at his or her convenience, if not during the actual visit.

Describe your history in writing.

Write out your history of pain, including when your pain began and what it's like—sharp, dull, constant, intermittent, provoked, unprovoked, etc. (For more information on the different degrees and qualities of pain, see Chapter 5. You can copy the self-questionnaire to use.)

Also describe your history of associated symptoms, especially those concerning bowels and bladder (since your digestive and urinary tracts are in your pelvis, sexual pain and organ pain often go together). If you had childhood issues with rashes, toilet training, or digestion, or if you've had orthopedic problems or injuries, include them as well.

You won't necessarily show this history to your physician, but do bring it with you. It will keep you focused during the visit and will help you answer your doctor's questions more easily.

Target three treatment goals.

Write out your three main goals of treatment, and share them with your doctor.

Here are some of the goals that our patients have expressed:

- comfortable intercourse

- ability to have sex on a regular basis

- no pain during or after sexual contact

- orgasms without pain afterward

- less worry about random sudden pain with sex

- stop bladder pain or bladder overactivity as a result of sex

- fewer muscle spasms during and after sex

- stop vulvovaginal burning and itching

- decrease hypersensitivity

- lessen the need to be overvigilant in avoiding pain in daily life

- prevent relapses

- reduce pain flare-ups

- feel free to date again

- improve a relationship

- wear jeans again

- wear underwear again

- feel comfortable sitting again

- feel normal again

- improve overall quality of life

- return to normal activities such as exercise

Take a survey of your pain.

Do this in advance so you can provide the information to the doctor. Links to these surveys are available in the Resources section of this book. We advise filling out the Numerical Pain Scale (NPS) *and* the Pelvic Pain Questionnaire (V–Q).

Bring paper and a pen.

Prepare a notebook and pen so you can take notes and write down any instructions during the visit.

Arrange to bring a support person with you if possible.

This person can serve you in many ways: by being an advocate for you, by offering you comfort during a potentially difficult experience, by taking notes on what the doctor says, by reminding you of questions, and by helping you remember afterward what the key points were.

Make sure to discuss ahead of time the role you want this person to play. Would you prefer them to sit quietly, to actively suggest questions, or to help you voice your concerns? Would you like them to accompany you into the examination room?

Ask administrative questions in advance.
Call ahead to find out from the office staff what the cost of the visit will be, how long it should take, and what insurance issues are involved. You don't want an unexpected bill to add to your stress.

Practice the discussion.
In the next section, we've offered you a couple of different scripts you might use for your first encounter with a doctor. Choose the one that seems most appropriate to your situation, adapt it to your own personality, and practice it a few times, alone or with a loved one. It's also fine to write something out and read it during the appointment.

Consider anti-anxiety medication.
If you're concerned about being so nervous that you won't be able to advocate for yourself effectively, ask another healthcare provider if taking a small dose of anti-anxiety medication before the visit might be appropriate.

Make yourself determined.
Affirm to yourself that you deserve good care, and remember that this is just the first step to getting it.

CREATIVE WAYS TO WORK WITH DOCTORS WHO ACCEPT INSURANCE

If a doctor accepts insurance, you may be only able to work with him or her in fifteen-minute increments, which won't be enough to diagnose and treat a sexual-pain condition. Here are some possibilities for working within that framework:

- Try to find a way to book several fifteen-minute appointments that the insurance company will accept.

- Consider working through a combination of emails, faxes, and personal appointments (but don't try to work things out by phone—that's always difficult for doctors).

- Offer to do some or all of the doctor's research.

- Help the doctor put together the team of specialists and support people that he or she might need to consult with, and organize the communication between your doctors (which will help you avoid getting disconnected care).

- Ask if the doctor can be your "home base" MD—the one who will coordinate your possibly complicated care, even if his or her knowledge base needs to be expanded.

STEP FOUR: MEET THE DOCTOR

Unless you have heard very good things about your doctor from other sexual-pain patients, we suggest you consider your first visit an opportunity to interview the doctor and to determine whether he or she will be able to work with you and treat you effectively. So many doctors are not willing or able to treat sexual pain—and many don't even realize that they aren't. You will need to be far more proactive than in any other type of medical situation—more proactive than you ever dreamed you had to be.

Here's how we suggest you handle the interview.

Your initial visit with the doctor will be much easier if you are in your street clothes rather than in an exam robe. So ask to see the doctor in the consulting room before disrobing for the exam. Explain that you understand this is not the normal procedure, that you expect only the usual fifteen-minute appointment, and that you are prepared to pay for a second fifteen-minute appointment, to be scheduled at another time, if the doctor is not able to both meet with you and examine you.

When the doctor arrives, we suggest you be both respectful and assertive. Even though you've brought written documents, don't give them to the doctor immediately; use them only for your own reference. Explain your pain history in your own words, and briefly state your goals for treatment. Then ask if the doctor has any experience with patients with your problem, and how comfortable he or she is with taking care of those patients.

As tactfully as you can, try to find out how experienced and well-educated the doctor is regarding your condition. You will have read the appropriate chapters in this book about your condition, so you can ask a few questions based on those chapters to see if your prospective MD knows even as much as you do. If you're not comfortable with his or her response, end the interview and continue with your search.

If the doctor says he or she has no experience, say something like the following:

Doctor, I'm taking this unusual step because I've been told by other practitioners that I have a sexual-pain condition that is not unusual, but that can be hard to treat. I want to be sure we're on the same page before I waste your time with further visits, and I'd like to ask your permission to talk to you about what I think might be going on with me, with the understanding that you're the doctor and that I defer to your expertise. I understand that your time is limited, and I'm happy to pay for this appointment and come back for another appointment so that this one stays within the time frame that you've allowed. But I'd like to use this time to talk with you, if that's alright with you. Do I have your permission to go ahead?

If the doctor doesn't agree to this request or insists on examining you before the two of you speak, we suggest that you simply leave. Do what you think is correct about paying or not paying for the appointment, but a doctor who is not willing to have a conversation with you about your situation is probably not a doctor who will treat your complex case with the care and attention and creativity that you need.

If the doctor agrees to continue, you can say something like the following, being careful to use the buzzwords we have emphasized.

I want to share with you some of the scientific material I've found about my condition, and to see what you think of it. I'm not trying to self-diagnose; I understand that only an MD is qualified to make a diagnosis. But I have done some scientific research—not pseudo-science, and not research on the Internet, which I realize is unreliable—but research in such juried medical and scientific journals as the American Journal of Obstetrics and Gynecology.

I've also found a book by an MD and a member of ACOG (American College of Obstetricians and Gynecologists) who suggests a medical approach to my condition. This is a medical approach, not an alternative approach, but it is one that many doctors aren't aware of, just because sexual pain isn't a big part of gynecology. So this is a specialized area, and I'm asking whether you would be willing to look at some specialized articles from standard medical journals to help you diagnose me and come up with a treatment plan. Would you be willing to consider that, and to at least look at the scientific-journal articles I've brought in, or perhaps also look at this book?

If your physician is open to looking at the recommendations in this book, continue with the visit. If your physician seems both inexperienced and unwilling to learn more, end the interview.

Again, it would not be unusual if you had to visit several physicians before finding someone who can offer you effective treatment. This may seem like a difficult task, but we want you to be prepared for the situation. You'll have to walk a fine line between compromising on a doctor who is not ideal and settling for a doctor who really can't help you.

STEP FIVE: UNDERGO AN EXAM

Once you've found a doctor you initially trust, your next step will be to undergo an examination. Here are some suggestions for how you can help the exam go as smoothly as possible, and some information for you about what the physician should be doing during the exam.

- Empty your bladder before the exam. If you feel very constipated, let the doctor know.

- If in the past you have had a great deal of pain triggered by certain parts of an exam, let the doctor know. Be as specific as you can, for example: "The speculum gives me severe pain, and I may end up pulling away," or "Having my clitoris touched with a finger may be too painful to me." If part of the exam cannot be completed, that is not your fault, but the fault of your sexual-pain condition. Do not ever submit to more than you can physically or psychologically handle, especially at the first exam. Future exams will be easier, and some steps may need to wait until then.

• Before the actual pelvic exam, your doctor should examine your gait, posture, back, hips, and abdomen, as each area may hold hints as to where your pain is coming from.

• When your doctor examines your pelvis itself, he or she will need to focus on several areas: skin, nerves, muscles, hips and joints, and organs. You'll be placed in the "lithotomy position," with your feet in stirrups and your bottom down at the edge of the examining table, so the doctor can see your vulva up close.

• The doctor needs to examine your vulvar surface with a magnifier (often a colposcope) to get a really good look. (You can recognize a colposcope because it looks like a binocular on wheels.)

• To evaluate your surface nerves and sensation, the doctor will need to use a cotton swab to find the areas of your vulva that are most tender.

• Your pelvic floor should also be examined. Your physician should cover his or her gloved finger with a nonirritating lubricant gel and insert it into your vagina, assessing each muscle area and connective tissue for tender points, tension, symmetry, and trigger points. It should be very systematic, with you giving feedback on what hurts.

• During the digital (finger) exam, your doctor also needs to evaluate the tenderness of the pudendal nerves, near the sides of the pelvis. When a normal pudendal nerve is touched, it creates a sensation similar to when your "funny bone" is touched. When the nerve is involved in your pain, touching it may cause sharp waves of pain to radiate to other areas of your pelvis or even to your back or hips.

- Finally, your doctor has to examine your pelvic organs—bladder, rectum, cervix, uterus, ovaries—feeling for abnormalities and tenderness.

- During these exams, your doctor will be taking wet smears of vaginal secretions and cultures to test for yeast and bacteria. He or she might also take a Pap test.

- If you are also getting a speculum exam, your doctor will use a small "opener" with lubricant to visually check the appearance of your vaginal canal and cervix.

We know that you can't exactly monitor the doctor to make sure that every one of these steps has been done, but you can follow him or her generally. A good initial exam for sexual pain takes about fifteen minutes, so if yours is five minutes or less, you can deduce that a few steps were left out. You can use your sense of how careful, thorough, and sensitive the exam is as another factor in deciding whether this doctor is right for you.

PAIN AS A CLUE

If your exam becomes painful at any point, tell your doctor, since this is significant information for the diagnosis. Stop the doctor if at any point the exam approaches a degree of pain that you can't bear. Keeping your muscles as loose as possible will help.

STEP SIX: DEVELOP A WORKING DIAGNOSIS AND A TREATMENT PLAN

After your exam is over, discuss the findings with your doctor in the consultation room if possible, since you'll feel far more empowered talking when you're fully dressed again. The discussion should begin with your doctor giving you a preliminary idea of what he or she thinks is causing your pain. It's fine if there's no diagnosis yet, as long as your doctor has specific plans for how to develop one.

Conceivably, time will run out before this part of the visit, so schedule a follow-up visit as soon as possible. Be aware that your doctor may need some time to review your history and tests before feeling comfortable diagnosing you. If your doctor believes more testing is needed, he or she should explain the plan. If necessary, take notes and email your understanding of the plan to the doctor's office for confirmation, or ask the doctor to give you a written version of the plan, to avoid confusion. Your doctor may well need to bring in consultations from other fields, including urology, orthopedics, neurology, dermatology, gastroenterology, and pain management.

Whenever the meeting continues, bring up your treatment goals. Your doctor's response to those goals will give you more information about whether you want to keep working with him or her. You should end either your first or your second visit with a treatment plan. Ask for as many details as you need to understand the plan, and be aware that it may be modified as further test results come back.

DOCTOR VISITS: DOS AND DON'TS

- Do keep track of your medical testing, and keep copies of everything.

➤

➤

- Do be punctual for every visit, and give twenty-four hours' notice for cancellations. Many doctors caring for chronic-pain patients save a lot of time for each appointment, so a late cancellation means the doctor is left with wasted time that another patient might have been able to use.

- Do be friendly and polite with the staff, bearing in mind that working at an office that cares for patients with chronic pain is very stressful for the support staff. A kind word will go a long way—they will remember and appreciate you.

- Don't blame the office staff for problems they can't help, such as insurance problems, doctors running late, costs of visits, and the like.

STEP SEVEN: MAKE YOUR DECISION

Once you've been through the consultation and perhaps also the exam, take some time at home to decompress. Then consider your response to the doctor. Was he or she attentive, optimistic, complete, upfront, open, empathetic? Or was he or she rushed, impersonal, overwhelmed, condescending, negative? Did he or she attribute your problems to your "catastrophizing" or to some other psychological cause?

If you decide that this is the right person for you to work with, reorganize your paperwork and review what you need to do. If you have received a treatment plan, does it make sense to you? You will need to take responsibility for this plan as well, obtaining the tests, consultations, and medications your doctor recommends. You are one-half of the partnership and will need to do your part if your treatment is to be successful.

If you decide that this isn't the right doctor for you, take a breath, give yourself a treat or a break—and then go back to the search process. It is perfectly normal to feel like giving up, but please don't. Once you find the right doctor, your condition will improve, so it's worth taking the time you need to find the right person.

EVALUATING YOUR DOCTOR: A CHECKLIST

As you're deciding whether to continue with the physician you've found, consider the following:

- ☐ Did your doctor seem to have enough experience treating sexual or vulvovaginal pain?

- ☐ Was your doctor open to new ideas?

- ☐ Was your doctor compassionate and caring?

- ☐ Did your doctor suggest that the problem was that you need to relax?

- ☐ Did your doctor suggest that the problem was primarily psychological?

- ☐ Did your doctor say there was nothing he or she could do to help? (If so, don't panic—there are other doctors who can help.)

- ☐ Was your doctor willing to do the needed research and to contact other doctors to help you, even if he or she doesn't yet know enough about your condition?

- ☐ Did your doctor have a positive attitude?

- ☐ Did your doctor leave you feeling hopeful that you can get better?

➤

➤
- ☐ Was your doctor honest about his or her limits?
- ☐ Did your doctor say that he or she was willing to work with you?
- ☐ Did your doctor say he or she is accessible to you between appointments?

STEP EIGHT: GET READY FOR FOLLOW-UPS

Prepare for follow-up visits by writing down any new symptoms you've had and new questions that arise. Prepare for testing by finding out all you can ahead of time, and perhaps bringing your advocate with you. We know that testing can be scary, but preparation should help.

We strongly urge you to get all your questions answered before any invasive or complicated tests, especially surgical procedures that require anesthesia. If necessary, get a second opinion. You want to make sure that there's no easier way to get the same information about your condition.

STEP NINE: CONSULT WITH SPECIALISTS

Use the same procedure to consult with specialists that we've suggested for selecting a gynecologist. Although it can be as difficult to find good specialists as it was to find the right gynecologist, caring doctors are out there, and you will eventually find them. Although you may need to make some compromises, specialists should also provide you with respect, time, and attention.

Be sure to ask how communication will occur between your consulting physicians and your "home base" doctor. Offer your help; for example, you might hand-deliver reports, if appropriate. Delays and uncoordinated care are common, and you want your next visit with your doctor to be as fruitful as possible.

STEP TEN: STAY POSITIVE

As we've said repeatedly, you may need to talk with many doctors over several months before finding the care that is right for you. While you're looking, there's a lot you can do to improve your sexual health, relieve stress, and gather your strength, through nutrition, good sleep, and appropriate exercise (for suggestions, see Chapter 4).

We know that finding the right doctor can be overwhelming. But the outlook is great when you do. Here's a message of hope from Stephanie, the patient we met in Chapter 1: "One thing that really helped me when I met with Dr. Coady was that she asked me what I wanted to call this," Stephanie says. "She said we can call it a 'project,' but I felt that sounded too clinical. So we agreed to call it an 'adventure.'"

4

BEGINNING
YOUR
HEALING

I used to do yoga . . . but when I had a pain flare-up, I'd have to stop—or sometimes, the yoga stretching might even set me off. Meditation gives me a lot of the same relaxation benefits as yoga, and it seems to be safer for my condition. It really helps me gather my energy and release stress—and when I'm coping with sexual pain, I need both.

—MARY, A TEACHER IN HER FORTIES

I find that work is very therapeutic for me. I am able to compartmentalize and shift into a different zone. Being of service to others is helpful to me, and it distracts me from my pain. . . . Another thing that helps me is to stay as physically active as I can. When I get home, I try not to stop moving for a while. I find that when I move my body, I am in less pain.

—BLAIR, A TEACHER IN HER EARLY FIFTIES

My daily pain journal allows me to get a perspective on my pain.
. . . The worst part of a flare-up is you never know when you will
feel better. If I'm having a pain flare-up and feel anxious because I
don't know how long it will last, I look at the pain journal, and it
reminds me that my flare-ups always calm down.

—KAREN, A FASHION DESIGNER IN HER LATE TWENTIES

WHETHER OR NOT you've yet found the physician of your choice, there is still a great deal you can do to support your own healing, both physically and emotionally. Indeed, because stress exacerbates pain, caring for yourself in all ways is crucial to recovery. In this chapter, we'll share some powerful healing strategies—for body, mind, and spirit—that you can begin using immediately.

HOW TO BEGIN YOUR HEALING PHYSICALLY

We've put together some suggestions for how to restore yourself physically and emotionally while you are seeking a doctor or while you are waiting for your medical treatments to take effect. For some of you, this advice might feel helpful. But for others, this advice may seem just like more restrictions and tasks in your already restricted, overwhelmed, and burdened life. Just choose what you feel comfortable with and only follow the advice that fits into your life. If it feels burdensome to you, then please do not add these recommendations to your regimen. You don't want to make your life harder than it already is. But if these suggestions seem helpful to you, by all means, incorporate them into your life, as they will improve your overall well-being.

Stop doing anything that hurts.

This may include having sex or exercising in your usual way. For many of us, exercise is a lifeline, and one of the worst aspects of sexual pain is having to give up the workouts and routines we normally rely on. Later in this chapter, we'll suggest some alternatives that you may be able to use if your usual workouts hurt or aren't possible for a while.

Many of us also find it difficult to accept, admit, or assert that we don't feel like having sex, but you really are allowed to say no, even to a beloved life partner, or to a more casual partner who you feel "deserves" to be satisfied. See Chapter 14 for types of sexual contact that can help you bypass some of the worst sources of sexual pain, so that if you choose, you can enjoy sexual pleasure. But don't feel you owe it to your partner or to yourself to risk any amount of pain, especially because what causes you pain might also delay your healing, or even set it back.

With this kind of condition, there's no such thing as "working through the pain," and your sexual pain won't go away if you push yourself through a workout routine or if you force yourself to have sex more often. We often say that "pain begets pain." There's no such thing as "getting used to it" when it comes to sexual pain, and continuing to do something that hurts is the equivalent of an athlete continuing to play after a major sports injury— you could very well make things worse, even permanently worse. Being gentle and good to yourself is the fastest way to come through this condition as quickly as possible, and in the best possible shape.

Promote genital wellness.

Avoid all potential toxins, including soaps, creams, and other topical treatments. Don't let any potential irritant touch your vulva or vestibule (the vaginal opening), especially benzocaine, alcohol, parabens, perfumes, and propylene glycol, which are in almost all over-the-counter remedies. Remember, even the gentlest soap is drying and is not needed there: the vagina and vestibule clean themselves constantly.

Wear very comfortable cotton underwear, well rinsed of laundry detergent, and change two or three times during the day, as opposed to wearing mini-pads, which cause sweating and may be more irritating. Use tampons without chemicals if you can tolerate a tampon, or else use only hypoallergenic, nonperfumed sanitary napkins. And to further avoid contact irritation, sleep without underwear or pants.

At least two to five times a day, apply some of the natural, irritant-free products listed below to the vulvar skin. This will help provide a barrier against the world and its rubbing, and will hydrate and combat dryness, which weakens the tissues. Make especially sure you use one of the following ointments (these are examples) as a coating before swimming in chlorinated pools.

- Aquaphor

- natural oils, such as olive, safflower, almond, coconut

- Nature's Gate Vitamin E Oil (contains grapeseed and safflower oils)

- Walgreen's Skin Oil with Vitamin E (contains safflower oil)

Alternately, if you're very sensitive, your physician can have a pharmacy compound other irritant-free oils. If you sweat a lot in the vulvar area, you may feel that powders are more comfortable, but most are irritating, so only use cornstarch in a light dusting if this is your choice.

Practice sleep hygiene.

Believe it or not, sleep is one of the key ways your body heals itself, and one of the best things you can do to alleviate your sexual pain is to get good, restful sleep. In fact, your pelvic floor muscles may only relax when you are in deep sleep, and only then can they get the blood flow they need.

If pain or anxiety about your condition is keeping you from sleeping deeply, talk to your physician about nonaddictive medications that might help you through this difficult time.

You can also make sure to create a sleep environment that will guarantee you the best night's rest. Everyone has her own preferences, so feel free to create your own ideal environment. But here are some sleep-hygiene basics that many people find helpful.

- a comfortable bed with a firm foam mattress that you use only for sleeping or sex

- a dark, quiet bedroom—no noise or light at bedtime

- a regular bedtime

- no sweets or stimulants for at least an hour (and possibly four to six hours) before bedtime

- no exercise for at least two hours before bedtime—it will actually wake you up

- if necessary, avoid electronic screens (including TV and computers) at least an hour before bedtime—the flickering light throws off your circadian rhythms

- a soothing fifteen- to sixty-minute bedtime routine, which might include a warm bath or another relaxing ritual, such as aromatherapy, meditation, or some other conscious way to let go of the troubles of the day

Nourish your nerves and your body.
Taking care of your nerves is a useful self-treatment for anyone with chronic pain, which always involves disordered nerves, at least to some extent. The supplements listed below will help restore your nerves to a healthier state.

- alpha lipoic acid
- magnesium
- vitamin B12
- thiamine

- vitamin D3
- folic acid (folate)
- omega-3 fatty acids
- acetyl-L-carnitine

Consider a low-dose, high-quality DHEA supplement, which, at 10mg to 25mg a day, balances hormones and decreases inflammation.

We also recommend general good nutrition as a key way to support your nervous system. Avoid caffeine, sugar, and high-starch/processed-flour foods: They rev up your system, make it harder to get restful sleep, and create stress that makes it harder for nerves to heal. If you must have caffeinated drinks, try to limit them to one or at most two cups a day; drink them in the morning or at least before your evening meal; and consume them only when also eating protein—never on an empty stomach. Try to consume processed-flour foods with protein so they won't cause your blood sugar to spike.

Try to have at least some protein every time you consume food. Regular consumption of protein will keep your blood sugar balanced and will relieve stress on your adrenals, which will give you more energy overall and will support your entire endocrine and digestive system. Ideally, you'll have some high-quality, low-fat protein every three hours or so. Think of choices such as yogurt, low-fat cheese, hummus, bean dip, almond or cashew butter, or a few nuts.

Look into the "anti-inflammatory diet," which limits red meat, wheat, and dairy and may help nerve inflammation (see the Resources section).

Eat plenty of fresh fruits and vegetables, especially dark-green vegetables such as kale, collard, chard, broccoli, and arugula.

Take a high-quality oral probiotic to balance your bowel and vaginal flora and to avoid infections.

Having said this, we know there are times when all you want in life is your favorite chocolate dessert or a big soothing plate of pasta. Be gentle with yourself as far as diet too. Eat as healthy as you can, but indulging yourself when you are in such pain is essential.

Increase oxygenation of your blood, brain, and nerves.
If you can keep up or even begin a regular aerobic exercise routine—brisk walking, swimming, rebounding (jumping on a miniature trampoline), or low-impact aerobics—that's terrific. If your condition makes that kind of exercise impossible, consider tai chi, Bikram or another form of yoga, or Pilates. All of these exercises are good for releasing stress and improving

sleep. And general fitness is important both to your overall health and to your sexual health, so to the extent that you can remain fit and active despite your sexual pain, you will be moving your healing forward.

If none of these activities are possible for you, see the boxed text "Relaxation Techniques" in this chapter. The deep breathing in each exercise will help oxygenate your blood and brain while also relieving stress.

Increase blood flow to your pelvic organs and tissues.

Exercise helps with this, so if possible, follow the suggestions in the previous section. We also advise trying qigong, a wonderful traditional Chinese medical exercise and art form that specifically focuses on increasing blood flow and flexibility in the pelvis, using gentle, conscious movements.

If you can't exercise normally—and especially if you're suffering from pelvic floor dysfunction (see Chapter 10) or orthopedically caused sexual pain (see Chapter 11)—we strongly recommend finding a physical therapist, which you can do even before you've found a doctor (see the Resources section for finding a physical therapist experienced in treating women with pelvic pain).

Balancing the pelvic floor muscles and mobilizing blood flow to your pelvic region are crucial for healing sexual pain. You may be astonished at how much progress you can make with your physical therapist even before you've found the right physician.

Massage is also an excellent way to improve blood flow to tissues and to release stress. You may need to look for a massage therapist who has experience working with people in pain. Your physical therapist should be able to help you find someone.

Try alternative methods of stress and pain management.

Stress has a number of negative effects on your body, mind, and spirit, and it's also been shown to worsen chronic pain. We know it's not easy, but every day that you can let go of some of the stress you're carrying is a day that you have taken one more step toward healing.

Healthy eating, restful sleep, gentle exercise, and massage are all excellent forms of stress release—as are the practices in the boxed text "Relaxation Techniques" and the gentle exercise routines mentioned above. At least once a week, give yourself a restful soothing treat—a spa day, some time in nature, your favorite funny movie, some time just to do nothing. Write this time into your schedule the way you would a doctor's appointment, because it's crucial to your recovery that you give your system some meaningful downtime.

Reflexology—a form of foot massage—is another excellent form of stress release, and one that may work better for you than traditional massage if you are in a lot of pelvic pain. Another option is hypnosis or self-hypnosis, which many women find to be an excellent form of pain management and a way to help with irritable bowel syndrome. Craniosacral therapy has also been effective for some of our patients.

We also highly recommend acupuncture, and many of our patients have found it extremely helpful in managing pain and promoting general health and well-being. Again, this is a proactive step you can take to improve your condition even before you have found a physician for medical treatment.

We don't recommend chiropractic treatments unless you have a practitioner who is really skilled in treating pelvic or sexual pain. If you are already working with someone you trust and who is helping you, terrific! Often though, chiropractors do not understand the needs of women with pelvic pain, and the wrong practitioner might very well make things worse.

RELAXATION TECHNIQUES

Here are four exercises to help you release stress and perhaps also ease your pain. Sometimes releasing stress also means releasing emotions, so you may find yourself feeling sad, angry,

➤

or anxious as you begin to let go. If you can, breathe through the feelings and allow them simply to flow through you, without responding to them. If you can't deal with what comes up, try a different technique or come back to the first one another day. Please don't judge yourself for any response you might have. Give yourself permission to feel however you actually feel, and to find the technique that works for you.

The first two techniques can be done even while on a conference call or in a meeting. All four can be done anywhere, including at work.

Although these relaxation techniques work for many people, they might not help you. If they don't, please don't feel that you've failed. These techniques don't work for everyone. There are many other ways to reduce your stress, so find the ones that are right for you.

HAND WARMING

This can be done anywhere, anytime, for as little as thirty seconds.

Visualize holding a warm cup of tea. Then think of a warm color that slowly surrounds your hands and wrists, seeping into your hands and deep into your palms, fingers, and wrists. Say to yourself, "My hands are getting warmer; my palms are getting warmer; my fingers are getting warmer; my wrists are getting warmer." This technique actually helps to recalibrate your autonomic nervous system (which regulates breathing, blood flow, and other automatic functions) and will improve your blood pressure, circulation, and pain responses. Ideally, you might try this technique once an hour for thirty to sixty seconds.

RELAXED BREATHING

This can be done anywhere, anytime, for as little as sixty seconds.

In any comfortable position, close your eyes and breathe in for a count of four and breathe out for a count of eight. Repeat four times, or as often as you like. Learn to use your diaphragm to breathe by placing your hand on your abdomen. As you breathe in, your abdomen should expand. As you breathe out, it should contract. Don't force your breath; simply allow it to float in and out.

PLEASANT IMAGERY

This can be done anywhere relatively private, including at work, for as little as three minutes.

Sit in a comfortable position, close your eyes, and breathe deeply. Let your mind float to a situation, place, or event you find particularly tranquil and peaceful: a beach, a mountaintop, a room in some familiar place—anything that makes you smile and feel safe. Allow each of your senses to awaken: see, hear, feel, smell, and taste the sensations of this place. Some people create added stress for themselves trying to find the "perfect" image. We suggest that you use any image that works for you, just as if you were daydreaming.

PROGRESSIVE MUSCLE RELAXATION

This can be done in any relatively private place, at home or at work. Ideally, allow five minutes for the exercise and five minutes to enjoy its benefits afterward.

In any comfortable position, take in and release a deep breath. Then tense and release each one of your muscle groups, in the following sequence: neck, eyes, shoulders, triceps, biceps,

> back, abdomen, butt, pelvic floor, thighs, calves, feet, and toes.
> After you tense each group of muscles, it will be more relaxed,
> so clench as hard as you can for about ten seconds, release, and
> then repeat once or twice. Ideally, complete this exercise once
> each day, and then give yourself about five minutes to simply
> sit, breathe, and relax.

HOW TO BEGIN YOUR HEALING EMOTIONALLY

In addition to taking special care of your physical self during this difficult time, it's extremely important to take care of your emotional self.

Find a therapist.

We can't stress this one too strongly. No matter what else is going right or wrong in your life, no matter what psychological strengths or mental health you have achieved, you will find it extremely difficult to manage the intense pain and psychological stressors of your sexual pain without an experienced therapist who understands the effects of chronic pain. Think of yourself as a soldier undergoing combat duty or as a survivor of a natural disaster. No matter what strengths you could bring to such a situation, you would likely need help in making it through.

Our bias is toward a therapist with some cognitive–behavioral training, because you will need support in coming up with day-to-day coping mechanisms, whether or not you're interested in long-term analysis of other issues. But the key is not the therapist's professional orientation but whether he or she is equipped to help people with chronic pain. That is a special area, and you need someone who specifically understands it.

If you're already seeing a therapist who's helping you with your condition, congratulations. If you're seeing a therapist who's helpful in other ways but is not willing or able to talk about immediate coping strategies, we suggest you find an additional therapist with pain management training while working with your current therapist on other issues. And if you're not seeing anyone, please, please start. After years of working with hundreds of patients in this field, both of us feel strongly that it is nearly impossible to survive the demands of a chronic sexual-pain condition without some kind of psychological support from a trained professional who understands what you're going through. Just as you wouldn't try to have a baby without a professional who is specifically trained in helping you deliver, so you shouldn't try to go through your sexual-pain journey without someone who understands the challenges of your condition.

By the way, as we have discussed earlier, attributing psychological causes to sexual pain is all too common, even among medical and mental-health professionals. Make sure that your therapist understands that your sexual pain is just as physical a condition as a broken leg or a diseased heart. While there may be a psychological component to every illness, you are not experiencing your condition because of your attitudes about sex, your strict upbringing, or any of the other urban myths out there. What you're going through has its roots in nerves, muscles, organs, and bones, and your therapist needs to understand that.

Use the Internet carefully.

There are many, many wonderful things about the Internet. If you want to go online to find a practitioner, a physical therapist, a hypnotist, or a massage therapist, we are delighted to hear it. But if you want to look for information about sexual pain, please don't. We regularly scan the Internet and are appalled at the poor quality of information, the extent to which physical conditions are referred to as psychologically based, and the sheer amount of misinformation on even the most reliable medical websites. You won't find good information online unless you know exactly where to look (we have some suggestions for you in the Resources section), and what you will find is likely to inspire self-doubt, self-blame, and shame—all the negative attitudes that may already be hurting you. Maybe at some point, good information will be widely available, but as of this writing, you're unlikely to find it online.

Likewise, although we recommend live support groups, we counsel against becoming involved in most of the chat rooms we have seen online. Many of them only seem to encourage what therapists call rumination and perseveration—obsessively thinking about your problem and continuing to talk about it in the same unchanging terms. We want to support your feelings; we believe you need to talk about your condition; and we'd love you to find other women with sexual pain with whom you can share experiences and advice, whether in person, by phone, or via email. There are also some newer professionally guided blogs that share helpful medical and psychological information. But we recommend avoiding chat rooms and blogs that reinforce helplessness and hopelessness, and leave you feeling negative and unsupported instead of optimistic, as you should be.

Be gentle with yourself.

If we could only give you one piece of advice to support you through your entire struggle with sexual pain, it would be "Be gentle with yourself." Sexual pain can be devastating. Its intensity is often overwhelming, both physically and emotionally. There will be times when you can do a great deal to make things better for yourself, and there will be times when you won't even have the energy to get out of bed. The best way through the hard times is to allow yourself to have them, to let yourself fall apart occasionally, and even to permit yourself the thoughts of suicide that virtually every woman in severe chronic pain considers, just as a way to assert control over her body and her life.

Being gentle doesn't mean giving up, and it doesn't mean giving in permanently to despair. Nor does it mean becoming a passive spectator of your own illness, waiting hopelessly for someone to come along and help you. Help is out there, but it is often hard to find, and you will need all of your physical and emotional resources to keep looking, and then to participate actively in your own treatment. The suggestions in this chapter are meant to support you, physically and emotionally, through all phases of your healing journey. They're meant to help you to care for yourself as fully and actively as possible when you can, and to let go and give yourself a break when you can't.

Every woman approaches her own healing differently, and so we want you to use the information in this chapter in the way that works best for you. You might want to adopt as many strategies as possible as soon as you can, or you might prefer a more gradual approach, choosing only one self-healing activity and getting used to its place in your routine before you even think about adding another. You might want to concentrate on physical approaches to healing—avoiding irritants, for example, or applying a soothing ointment—or you may be more focused on psychological or spiritual therapies.

As we've said, there also may be times when you don't feel up to doing anything at all. At one particularly emotional therapy session, Karen told Nancy, "I remember you told me that taking a break from the world and staying in bed all day is just something I have to do sometimes. I feel so much better remembering that, because I used to think that when I laid in bed all day, I was giving in to my pain. And then, by the end of the day, when I felt I hadn't accomplished anything, I always felt anxious. Your reassurance means a lot to me."

Strange as it may seem, for many women, an essential coping mechanism is to imagine suicide as a possible way out. If you find yourself continually preoccupied with killing yourself and making active plans to do so, we urge you to find a loved one and to go to your local emergency room immediately. Suicide is not an alternative if you believe, as we do, that a joyous, fulfilling life awaits you, even if your condition can't be totally cured. But if you simply imagine suicide as a possible way out of a life of pain, take heart. Virtually every woman who struggles with sexual pain spends some time with suicidal thoughts, not as an actual intention, but as an imagined escape route, a fantasy.

"When I first experienced the pain, I was suicidal," admits Jessie, the businesswoman we met in Chapter 1. "If someone had said to me, 'You will have to live like this the rest of your life,' I would have thrown myself in front of a bus."

Kate, the former film producer from Chapter 2, actually felt upset at the thought that she would probably not commit suicide. "I can tell you when I got the most depressed," she says. "I came home one day after a therapy session and was sobbing. It had dawned on me that I could never really kill myself. And that was the worst thing—knowing that killing myself was no longer an option for me. Because now I had no way out of my pain."

Before her revelation, however, Kate says she often thought about committing suicide as a way of escaping her torturous pain. But she knew she couldn't do it, because, as she says, "I am a perfectionist, and I didn't want to make a mistake and end up on a ventilator. And I am also really terrified that tomorrow I suddenly might not be in as much pain, or as depressed, and if I killed myself, I would miss that possibility."

Other women have told us they fantasized about suicide but then thought of how their children or other loved ones might be affected; that spiritual thoughts or religious faith pulled them back; or that a sense of mission and purpose about their life's goals kept them anchored in the world. While we would not wish on anyone the pain and despair that lead to suicidal thoughts, we do affirm both that having the choice—even in your thoughts—can be empowering, and that it can be even more empowering to connect with what in life means the most to you. When you have to critically assess and evaluate whether you want to remain alive, you gain a deeper appreciation of what is truly important to you. And parts of your life that may not have seemed so important take on much greater significance. For example, being home for your child when he or she comes home from school or holding hands with your partner while watching TV at one point in your life may not have seemed so significant. But when you are evaluating whether suicide is an option, you begin to realize how these aspects of your life that you once took for granted are actually monumental moments.

Please remember that it is *essential* that you share suicidal thoughts with a therapist or someone you trust. It is destructive and dangerous to keep these thoughts and feelings to yourself.

Whatever your thoughts and feelings about any of these issues, we urge you to stay connected to your support system, to be gentle and compassionate with yourself, and to hold on to the possibility that help and effective treatments are out there. If you are having these suicidal fantasies, you need to know that they are completely normal—but we urge you not to simply sit with them.

Here are some things you can do to help yourself feel better and get better. Find ways of talking with your loved ones, look for other women who have shared your experience, and work with a therapist who can help you come to terms with these feelings. If you are a single woman, please don't assume that sexual pain has disqualified you from finding anyone. Even if you have chosen a single lifestyle, healing your sexual pain is still critical, because it may worsen and become a complicated pain syndrome. See Chapters 14 and 15 for suggestions on how to move forward—even with sexual pain.

Listen to yourself.

There is so much you can do at every point to begin, continue, and support your healing. But your healing journey will probably not proceed on a smooth path or in a straight line. We urge you to be proactive and gentle with yourself; to take action and to give yourself a break; to be disciplined and indulgent.

Ultimately, your best guide along your healing journey is your own inner voice. That voice may be hard to make out through the pain and despair, but we promise you, it is always there. Give yourself the time and space to listen, and you will hear it.

PART TWO

UNDERSTANDING THE PROBLEM

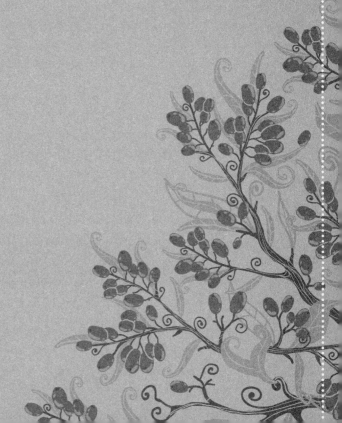

5

.....

FIGURING

OUT

WHAT YOU

HAVE

I never experienced this kind of pain before. I felt fine one day and the next day I was in severe pain. The scariest thing was that I had no clue what was wrong with me. I'm not sure which was worse, the pain or the not knowing what was wrong with me.

—MARY, A TEACHER IN HER FORTIES

NE OF THE most difficult aspects of sexual pain is not knowing exactly what's wrong. You know it hurts—sometimes beyond anything you've ever experienced or could imagine—but the pain may seem mysterious, as well as overwhelming. Indeed, part of what makes it so overwhelming is not being able to isolate, identify, or classify it—especially if, like most of the women we treat, you've been given an inaccurate diagnosis, conflicting diagnoses, or no diagnosis at all.

Don't worry: Help is on the way! In this chapter, we'll show you how to identify specific symptoms so that you can recognize which conditions you might be suffering from. And you will gain a wider understanding of what pain actually is. You can then go on to read about specific conditions (in Chapters 6 through 13).

IDENTIFYING THE PROBLEM

Let's be very clear: We are not asking you to diagnose yourself. Only a knowledgeable physician can make a true diagnosis, and it's important that you work respectfully with anyone who offers you treatment.

However, as we've explained in Chapter 3, it might take you a while to find someone who can treat you properly. When you do find that person, he or she may need your help in getting up to speed on the latest research. Meanwhile, you need answers about what may be going on with your body, so that you can understand what's happening to you, and so that you can have some idea of what to expect. In this chapter, we'll help you figure out what conditions you might have.

We say "conditions," in the plural, because frequently, the women we treat are suffering from more than one condition causing sexual pain. As a result, you may need to read more than one of the chapters in Part 2. Sexual pain begins in the pelvis—and everything in the pelvis is connected to everything else.

The pelvis is the area of the body that extends from your lower abdomen in front and from your spine in back, down to your upper legs, forming a basin-shaped hollow frame at your hips. It supports all of your internal organs—including your kidneys, liver, intestines, stomach, uterus, ovaries, and bladder—and provides attachment to the muscles and bones of your legs.

The vulva and sexual organs are also contained within the pelvis, which is why sexual pain is such a complex condition, with one condition easily morphing into many others. Skin pain can go deeper, affecting nerves that lie well below the surface. Orthopedic pain can cause pelvic muscles to spasm; disorders of the bladder can affect adjacent organs. We have seen many cases of untreated vestibulodynia (a condition in the vestibule, or entry, of the vagina) progress to cause pain and spasming in the pelvic floor muscles, which then causes bladder pressure and pain, or pudendal nerve compression and pain. A problem that was localized in one area now extends into several.

Luckily, the reverse is also true: Treating one condition can often benefit another condition. That's why finding good medical assistance is so crucial—and why you have so much reason for hope once you find it.

So let's get started. In this chapter, we'll take you through three steps.

Understanding Chronic Pain

Whatever your specific disorder, it's likely you've been suffering from a type of chronic pain—one of the least understood conditions in modern medicine, and one of the hardest for any patient to bear.

Intense chronic pain is unlike any other experience. It has the ability to undermine our human abilities to analyze, qualify, and predict, reducing us to primal animal selves that know only one thing: *This hurts so much I can't believe it will ever stop—and I can't think, feel, or want anything until it does.* If you are able to visualize what's happening in your body and to understand the causes, you can at least get some perspective on your pain. Your ultimate goal, of course, is to vastly reduce and perhaps even eliminate the pain entirely—but meanwhile, you will find it empowering to know more about what's happening to you.

Identifying Symptoms and Assessing Pain

We'll share with you a basic pain questionnaire that's used by medical personnel to evaluate pain and to assess how it might be changing over time. This is a terrific way to see how treatment actually is making a difference.

We'll also provide you with a simple questionnaire to help you identify and organize your symptoms.

Identifying Possible Conditions

Once you've identified your symptoms, we'll help you figure out which conditions you might have—and which chapters to read. While this is no substitute for an actual physician's diagnosis, it will give you some information about what might be going on with you, and it will provide a good starting place when you do find the right doctor.

WHAT IS PAIN?

The medical definition of pain is deceptively simple. Pain is an unpleasant feeling carried by your nerves (neurons) to your brain as the result of an actual or potential injury. Your neurons are electrically excitable cells that carry information to your brain by means of chemical and electrical signaling.

In other words, when you are injured—or when your body is being stressed in a way that might produce injury (such as overexertion, exposure to heat, or some other possible danger)—your neurons register the sensation and pass the message along to your brain. Looked at in its most positive light, pain is nature's way of telling us there's a problem, so that we can avoid danger and repair injuries when they begin.

Even with this simple definition, pain has two aspects: 1) the physical sensation, and 2) the mental and emotional interpretations of it. To take another very simple example, we might feel the ache of our muscles as we lift a weight or engage in some other vigorous exercise, but we distinguish between this minor pain, which we recognize as healthy, and the more intense and potentially dangerous pain of a torn ligament or broken bone. Our judgment of when pain is excessive and when it's dangerous is an integral part of our experience of pain.

Anticipating pain can make it worse, and so can worrying about it. If you know that the pain you feel while running is a temporary side effect of exertion, you can more easily ignore it. If you're afraid that you've injured yourself or might be having a heart attack, you have to pay attention. In the same way, when you feel various types of sexual pain, you may experience the pain differently, depending on whether you know what it is, whether you feel you have control over making it stop, or whether you anticipate that it may become worse. Pain isn't fixed, it's fluid, and it's different for each of us—which sometimes makes it hard to talk about, to get others to take it seriously, and to explain to a physician.

As you've seen in previous chapters, your sexual pain is a real condition with identifiable physical causes. Sometimes it is an absolute—a condition that comes and goes on its own terms, impervious to your efforts to manage it (though we believe that with the right treatment, you can do a great deal to overcome the pain and perhaps eliminate it entirely). Sometimes, your psychological state can make a difference, which is why in Chapter 4 we recommended meditation and other psychological approaches, along with some physical treatments.

In all cases, we believe, knowledge is power. Getting to know your pain is often the first step to defeating it.

Referred Pain

A confusing phenomenon known as referred pain complicates the matter still further. Referred pain is when the nervous system interprets incorrectly and transfers pain from its actual source to another location. You might have a hip injury, for example, but feel the pain in your knee. If you have temporomandibular joint disorder (TMJ), a disorder of the jaw, you might experience your jaw pain as headache. People with organ disorders may experience their problems as a backache, stomachache, or indigestion instead of accurately locating their pain in the kidney, appendix, or gallbladder. When sexual pain is referred, it becomes harder to diagnose—though once you and your physician understand the source of the problem, it can be treated just as well as pain with a more obvious source.

Generalized Pain

Another phenomenon is generalized pain, in which you experience your pain as radiating throughout a whole region of your body—even though, medically speaking, your pain has only a single source. Again, this type of pain may be harder to interpret, but when it is understood, it can be treated.

PAIN TRIGGERS

Pain can have an immediate trigger, such as an injury—you twist your ankle, cut your finger, or bump your head. It can also be triggered by illness, such as when a bad flu makes you ache all over. Psychological conditions can also cause pain, such as when grief makes your chest ache, or when shock feels like an actual blow to the stomach.

Also, pain sometimes develops without an easily identifiable trigger (though often, we can figure it out in retrospect). Unfortunately, much of sexual pain falls under this category. Since you're used to pain having specific physical causes, the apparently unprovoked nature of much sexual pain can be bewildering, even terrifying. Despite its physical source in your skin, nerves, muscles, bones, organs, hormones, and/or immune system, sexual pain might indeed flare up unprovoked, which is one of its most frightening and disturbing aspects. This unprovoked aspect can make sexual pain more complicated to treat than other types of pain, but effective treatments do exist, so again, don't give up hope. Once you and your doctor understand the problem, help is there.

THRESHOLDS OF PAIN

Your pain threshold is the point at which you begin to feel pain. If someone gives you a playful tap on the arm, for example, you would not normally feel pain. But if someone gives you a serious punch, you would feel pain. The boundary between "mildly uncomfortable" and "painful" is your pain threshold.

Pain thresholds vary enormously among individuals, based on a variety of factors, including genetics, prenatal experience, infancy and early childhood pain, general health, and training. Pain thresholds can also vary for a single individual, and are likewise based on a variety of physical and psychological factors. Anger and adrenaline rushes famously raise the pain threshold, so that athletes, dancers, and people in emergency situations have been known to sustain injuries they didn't feel until later. Being in labor also increases the pain threshold, so women in childbirth are capable of sustaining pain they could not bear at other times.

Also, orgasm and stimulation in the G-spot raise your pain threshold. So if you can figure out how to get yourself aroused (with or without a partner) and experience orgasm in ways that don't involve pain, you will actually be improving your condition!

Depression, by contrast, decreases the pain threshold. Pain thresholds also remain lower than normal for several months or even years after detoxification from methadone and heroin. If chronically used, opioid painkillers can also lower your pain threshold, which is one reason we recommend avoiding them when you can. A condition known as fibromyalgia, which we'll consider in Chapter 13, also decreases pain thresholds, in addition to increasing sensitivity to cold and heat.

Prolonged chronic pain itself can also decrease your pain threshold. In other words, being in pain makes you increasingly more sensitive to pain. And if nerves in the genital area are injured, that area may have a lowered pain threshold, making it unusually sensitive to pain.

TYPES OF PAIN

There are several categories of pain. This section will help you identify which category or categories yours falls into. It will also help you get a better understanding of how pain works.

Acute vs Chronic Pain

A key distinction for understanding pain is acute versus chronic pain. Until you encountered chronic sexual pain, you may have experienced only acute pain. You may be tempted to view one kind of pain in terms of the other, but acute pain and chronic pain are actually two separate biological conditions. They are experienced differently, they respond to treatment differently, and they even operate via two different types of neural processing. Once you understand this, a lot of the formerly mystifying aspects of your chronic pain begin to make sense.

If you've been suffering from sexual pain for three to six months or more, your pain is primarily chronic. But since you and most of the people you know are more used to acute pain, it can be useful to contrast them.

ACUTE PAIN

Acute pain is self-limiting—usually, even if you don't do anything to make it better, it has a natural end in sight. Its function is to protect—usually to warn of tissue damage—and it's typically the symptom of some type of disease or response to an injury.

CHRONIC PAIN

Although chronic pain may fluctuate, there may be no spontaneous natural end in sight (though with the treatment we are encouraging you to find, it can be helped). As far as we know, most chronic pain has no function: It's a biological process gone haywire. Instead of being the warning of a potential disease process, it *is* a disease process: The nerves are not functioning the way they are supposed to, and as a result, they keep sending pain signals.

There are three ways to understand why chronic pain occurs, and to help you understand the anatomy of the nervous system, refer to illustrations 5-1 and 5-2:

- damage to the peripheral nervous and/or autonomic nervous system

- damage to the central nervous system

- a condition involving damage to two or three systems and/or to the interaction between them

Chronic pain resulting from nerve damage can be either constant or paroxysmal (in bursts), and it's most often described as burning, electric, tingling, itching, or shooting. Unlike most acute pain, it is not highly responsive to opioids (painkillers) or nonsteroidal anti-inflammatory drugs (NSAIDs; pain relievers such as aspirin and ibuprofen). It also has its own unique set of psychological side effects: depression, anxiety, hopelessness, despondency, lowered self-esteem, and a sense of isolation.

One of the challenges of chronic pain is its tendency to become "hard-wired" into the system, as though your neural pathways simply become used to transmitting unremitting pain signals. Because your nervous system is large and complex, and because it's all so interconnected, damage in one area may morph into more extensive malfunctioning in the central nervous system. That's why it's crucial to act quickly to get help with chronic pain: The longer you struggle with it, the harder it becomes to eradicate.

In medicine, there's a saying, "pain begets pain"—and this is particularly true of chronic pain. However, this same neuroplasticity (that is, the ability to rewire our brains in different ways) may also give us the ability to overcome pain that was once believed to be impervious to treatment. A lot of great new research is now focusing on the brain's ability to reduce or even eliminate pain by rewiring itself in this positive way.

Somatic vs Visceral Pain

There are two other classifications of pain.

One is somatic pain, which comes from the skin, muscles, ligaments, tendons, and fascia (a type of connective tissue) and deep tissues, and which is transmitted by peripheral nerves. Somatic pain tends to be what doctors refer to as "well localized"—that is, you experience it as located in a very specific place. It is generally constant; it is typically described as sharp, aching, throbbing, or gnawing; and it can be acute or chronic.

The other is visceral pain, which comes from the internal organs and is transmitted mostly by the autonomic nervous system. Visceral pain tends to feel more vaguely distributed throughout the body or a region of the body. It may come in short, sharp bursts (called paroxysms) and is usually described as deep, crampy, squeezing, or colicky. It may also be acute or chronic.

CROSS-TALK: WHEN SOMATIC AND VISCERAL PAIN ARE CONFUSED

To make diagnosis and treatment all the more complicated, we now know from recent research that the somatic and visceral nerves "cross-talk" in the lower spinal cord. (We have depicted part of the nervous system of the pelvis in illustration 5-1 with the pudendal nerve representative of the somatic nerves and the sympathetic plexus representative of the visceral nerves.) As a result, pain can be interpreted wrongly by the brain as coming from a skin or muscle area when it is really resulting from a problem in an organ. Elsewhere in the body, organ pain is kept quite separate from the pain of muscles, skin, and fascia. But in the lower spinal cord supplying the pelvis, these two types of pain get easily mixed up. Incredibly, the skin or muscle area in pain may then change: For example, with endometriosis pain in the organs, spinal cord signals may cause pelvic floor muscles to grip and increase their tension in ways impossible for you to consciously overcome. The problem may then spread to surrounding muscles, causing buttock or lower-back pain.

This is known as the visceral–somatic reflex (VSR). VSR is responsible for the complexity of sexual and pelvic pain, sometimes making it difficult to know which systems are the pain's source, and sometimes requiring us to direct treatment efforts in multiple directions.

Sexual Pain

Sexual pain has its own unique quality as well: Some of our brain's pain centers, as depicted in illustration 5-2, may overlap with the centers for sexual sensation, arousal, and orgasm. Deborah speculates that perhaps that is why sexual pain becomes such an intense, total-body, and deep pain experience—just as orgasm is also such a total-body, deep sensory experience. Sexual pain may be more profound and totalizing than, say, pain in the arm or leg, since the nerve fibers meant to transmit pleasure now transmit pain.

Again, we don't want you to lose hope. If you've been suffering for only a short while, act quickly to get help, because your speedy response can make a big difference. If you've been struggling with chronic pain for several months or more, we invite you to dig deep for additional reserves of

Illustration 5-1.

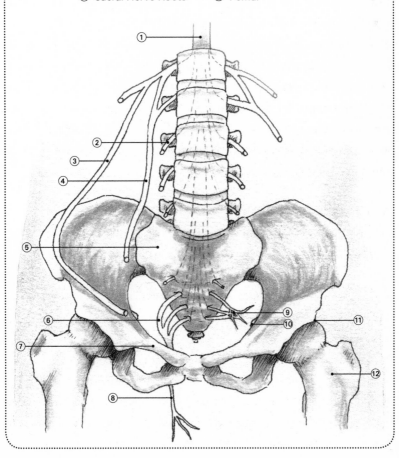

**THE PERIPHERAL AND AUTONOMIC
NERVOUS SYSTEMS**

① Lumbar Spine   ⑦ Pubic Bone
② Nerve Roots   ⑧ Pudendal Nerves
③ Ilioinguinal Nerve   ⑨ Sympathetic Plexus
④ Genitofemoral Nerve   ⑩ Ischial Spine
⑤ Sacrum   ⑪ Hip Joint
⑥ Sacral Nerve Roots   ⑫ Femur

patience. You can be helped—but it will probably take longer than it would have if your intervention had come earlier. Be prepared for a longer fight, but know that it can ultimately be successful—and don't give up.

THE PERIPHERAL NERVOUS SYSTEM

The peripheral nervous system is composed of all the nerves and ganglia (nerve cell bundles) outside the brain and the spinal cord (see illustrations 5-1 and 5-2).

The main nerve of the vulva is the pudendal nerve. Its branches carry sensation to the brain from the vulva and the pelvic floor (the set of muscles in your pelvis that supports all your organs).

If you're feeling sexual pain, your pudendal nerve may have been damaged at any one of a number of places: from the point it exits your lower spine at the sacrum, through one of its main branches that extend throughout your pelvis, or in one of the very tiny fibers that end at the skin of your vulva. No matter where along this long path your pain actually originates, you are likely to feel it as if it's coming from those vulvar tissues, where the tiny ends of the nerve are located.

What Causes Peripheral Nervous System Pain?

Chronic pain in the peripheral nervous system may be due to peripheral sensitization. There are a lot of ways your peripheral nerves can become overly sensitized, so that they send "extra" pain messages to your brain. When your nerves become injured, ill, damaged in some way, and are not functioning properly, we call this condition a "neuropathy," and the pain "neuropathic."

Remember, in acute pain, the pain messages represent an injury, illness, or specific cause, and the nerves are functioning appropriately. But in many types of chronic pain, the pain messages come from overly sensitive, injured peripheral nerves that have become hyperreactive. Their pain messages are not an alert to the brain that something is wrong—they're evidence that the nervous system isn't working properly.

So how can the peripheral nervous system misfire and make mistakes in the pain messages that it tries to transmit?

- The nerve endings themselves can be injured to varying degrees, from mild to severe. This may cause them to send inaccurate impulses—that is, inaccurate information about your sensations. In other words, they send pain signals saying *Something hurts!*—even when there is no reason for anything to hurt. As a result, you feel pain—but no scan or x-ray can make visible the cause of your pain.

- Sometimes the problem lies with the tissues surrounding the peripheral nerves. These tissues might "confuse" the nerves by compressing them, releasing toxic chemicals around them, or otherwise "fooling" them into believing there is a problem—and therefore causing them to send a pain signal to the brain.

- Sometimes the nerves and the tissues are "confused" into believing there is an intruder. They are affected by a kind of autoimmune response known as neurogenic inflammation—a chemical cascade designed to neutralize the virus, the bacteria, or the physical object they believe is threatening the tissue. Of course, there is no such intruder. The inflammatory response includes mast and other immune cells, which release their own array of signaling chemicals: cytokines, neurokines, substance P, and histamine, which signal more cells to come to the area to do the same. This is part of what we call the inflammatory cascade. This cascade inflames the peripheral nerves, causing them to send pain messages to the brain. We think this is what occurs in vestibulodynia (see Chapter 8).

- After a genuine injury, the nerves may "memorize" pain signals or become "hardwired" in a particular way to continue to send them, even when the surrounding tissues have healed and are no longer damaged or in danger.

- A tissue chemical known as nerve growth factor (NGF) might inappropriately trigger an overgrowth of nerves in a particular area, such as the clitoris or vestibule of the vagina. All these extra nerves are unusually sensitive and can react to even neutral or pleasant stimuli by sending pain signals.

Any or all of these factors can create peripheral sensitization, so that pain signals are sent for no apparent reason. Neuropathic pain may also lower your pain threshold, meaning that you feel more pain for lesser causes.

THE AUTONOMIC NERVOUS SYSTEM

The autonomic nervous system is the part of the nervous system that regulates breathing, heartbeat, digestion, and other "automatic" functions that we don't consciously control but that are crucial to staying alive. The visceral nerves are part of this system. Our pelvic organs—ovaries, uterus, bladder, and bowels—operate within this framework, which means that the autonomic nervous system is involved in reproduction, menstruation, urination, and defecation. As a result, disorders in the autonomic nervous system can have complicated, subtle, and far-reaching effects on our pelvic organs and their functions (especially the bladder and bowel) and can shape our specific experience of pain (see Chapter 12).

What Causes Autonomic Nervous System Pain?

Chronic pain or dysfunction based in the autonomic nervous system is called autonomic neuropathy, dysautonomia, or small fiber neuropathy. Chronic pain or dysfunction based in the autonomic nervous system is variously called autonomic neuropathy, dysautonomia, and small fiber neuropathy. Recently, we are recognizing that a portion of women with chronic vulvar pain, also known as vulvodynia, who have diffuse burning pain that feels like it is coming from the vulvar skin, are suffering from abnormalities in these small autonomic fibers that run in their nerves. Damage to these nerves is often seen in people with diabetes, in which abnormal small nerves in the feet send painful burning sensations to the brain in a condition known as diabetic neuropathy. In the vulva, the causes of this neuropathic pain may be diabetes, or autoimmune, infectious, toxin-related, or genetic conditions. Chapter 9 will give you more information about testing for autonomic causes of painful sex.

THE CENTRAL NERVOUS SYSTEM

The central nervous system is the body's command center: the brain and the spinal cord, which organize and integrate the information received from the peripheral and autonomic nervous systems. The spine holds long columns of nerves that are bundled together like fiber-optic cables and that transmit information to and from the brain. All sorts of information reach the brain: *Hot! Cold! Soft! Feels good!*

Pain signals are sent to several areas that are primarily designed to receive and then redistribute those signals to other parts of the brain that add consciousness, emotional color, and importance to the primary experience of pain.

Think for a moment what would happen if our bodies were not organized this way. There are some people, for example, who are born without the capacity to feel pain. No matter how badly they are injured, a rare autonomic nerve disorder keeps the pain signals from ever reaching their brains. As a result, they're at great risk, since they have no way of registering bodily danger or distress.

On the other hand, as we have seen, the emotional color and interpretation of pain matter enormously, since we discount or even welcome some types or degrees of pain. Some of us endure the pain of having our legs waxed or our hair dyed in the belief that the end result will be worth it. We might enjoy the pleasant ache of a strenuous workout or a vigorous massage.

Illustration 5-2.

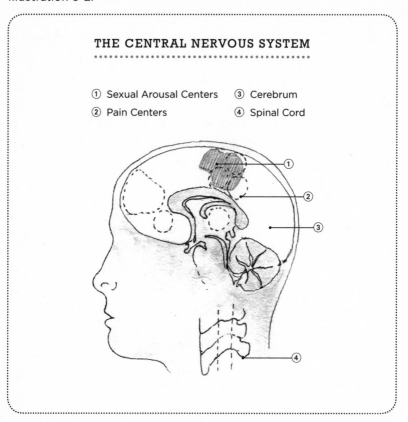

THE CENTRAL NERVOUS SYSTEM

① Sexual Arousal Centers   ③ Cerebrum

② Pain Centers   ④ Spinal Cord

Our brain helps us distinguish between these types of pain and others that might signal the need for action to make the pain stop. And of course, some people can't or won't tolerate these types of pain, seeking gentler beauty treatments and less-painful workouts.

So when our central nervous system is working well—when the brain and spine are properly organizing, transmitting, and interpreting nerve impulses and pain signals—we are getting useful information that helps us make important decisions: *Don't stop the masseur kneading our back. Do stop the four-year-old who's kicking us in frustration.* The problem comes when our central nervous system makes a mistake—and particularly, when it becomes oversensitized. Then, unfortunately, the pain can be unbearable.

What Causes Central Nervous System Sensitization?

When she first came to see us, our patient Elaine had been in pain for eight years due to fibromyalgia and vestibulodynia. "I'm a really stoic person, and I don't complain easily," Elaine told us soon after she came into the office. "But having this kind of pain that's centralized in my nervous system is agonizing, like constant torture." As Elaine describes it, "What an ordinary person might experience as pain is magnified about a hundred times for me."

In centralized pain disorders, pain is magnified in three ways. First, the nerves in the spinal cord transmit amplified pain impulses to the brain. Second, the special pain centers that initially receive those impulses are already primed or sensitized—overly ready to turn up the volume on even the slightest trace of pain. And third, at the same time, the parts of the nervous system that are supposed to inhibit pain (the parts we use to tolerate the bumps and bruises of everyday life) aren't working the way they're supposed to. So parts of the central nervous system are turning up the volume—and the equipment that's supposed to turn it down isn't working.

As a result, women who have pain disorders like Elaine's often hurt so much all over that the contact of soft clothing on their skin is intolerably agonizing. Unlike pain that is caused by an obvious physical injury, this category of pain seems to come out of nowhere and to intensify for no apparent reason. When there is no evidence of a recognizable pain-causing factor, the pain itself becomes the disease.

The following is a more specific breakdown of the factors that can cause centralized pain. Again, you might be suffering from just one of these factors, or several of them may be interacting.

- When the cascade of inflammatory chemicals creates sensitization and/or overgrowth among peripheral nerves, the spinal nerves may also change in response. These nerves feed back to the vulva through the pudendal nerve, creating a feedback loop that might trigger the pelvic muscles to spasm as well. This is the visceral–somatic reflex we talked about earlier.

- As they enter the spinal cord to become bundled into "fiber-optic cables," nerves sometimes inappropriately cross-talk with other nerves entering the spine at the same place. Somehow, these nerves get their "wires" crossed and send the brain incorrect messages, which get processed as intense chronic pain.

- In addition, the "fiber-optic bundles" can be compressed anywhere along their lengthy course. Such injuries can cause pain signals to be sent as if from the place where the nerve fiber ends. In other words, your pudendal nerve might be compressed near your spine, or a back injury may compress part of the spinal cord holding the fibers supplying the genitals. Significantly, you will feel the pain not at its true source, but where the nerve ends—in the skin of your clitoris and vulva.

- The brain is also supposed to send nerve impulses down to different levels of the spinal cord to inhibit incoming impulses of pain and other sensations traveling up to the brain. If this system makes mistakes, too many pain sensations will enter the brain.

- Nerve centers in the brain itself may incorrectly process pain messages, especially if you suffer from depression.

Unfortunately, centralized chronic pain can add to the pain you experience from the other specific causes of your particular condition. Even when your other conditions are treated effectively, your nervous system might continue to behave in a disordered way, causing the ongoing sensation of pain for no apparent reason. For example, the skin condition lichen sclerosus (discussed in Chapter 6) may be healed by applying ointments to the surface of the skin. But even after the skin is normal again, the underlying nerves might continue to send burning and itching pain signals to the brain, which inappropriately processes the signals, perpetuating the pain. In this case, it's not enough just to treat the skin—we also have to treat the nervous system.

And, as we have seen, the longer the nerves have been sending chronic pain signals, the longer it may take to calm them down, to desensitize them, and to reduce or eliminate the pain.

Another painful aspect of centralized pain is the "aftersensations" and residual pains that occur after a touch or other pain trigger; these pains can reverberate for days, long after the initial stimulus is over. This happens frequently with sexual pain, so that even a light sexual touch (let alone rubbing or intercourse) might create pain that continues long after the touch has ended. In some cases, even the pressure of wearing underwear, pantyhose, or jeans—or simply the act of sitting—creates this type of reverberating pain.

Types of Pain Associated with Central Sensitization

If you have central sensitization, you may be subject to any or all of these unusual types of pain.

ALLODYNIA

This is pain caused by a stimulus that normally does not cause pain, such as a light touch. If you've noticed that even putting on your underwear causes intense pain in your clitoral region, for example, you're suffering from allodynia.

HYPERALGESIA

This is increased sensitivity to a stimulus that would normally be considered minimally painful. For example, normally, if you're lightly scratched by a fingernail, that would cause mild pain. But if part of your body is suffering from hyperalgesia, a scratch in that region would be excruciatingly painful.

HYPERESTHESIA

This is increased sensitivity to sensory stimulation, sometimes resulting in pain. For example, you might experience with extra intensity a bright light, a loud noise, or a thick scratchy sweater—so much intensity that you actually feel pain. If you're suffering from hyperesthesia, you and the people around you may write off your responses as "being too sensitive." In fact, your nervous system has indeed made you "too sensitive"—but it's a disorder of your central nervous system, not a psychological response.

AVOID OPIOID PAIN MEDICATIONS

If you're in severe chronic pain, it can be tempting to reach for a painkiller, any painkiller—especially if your physician has prescribed it and assured you that it's okay. But watch out. An increasing amount of scientific evidence, backed up by clinical experience, suggests that opioid painkillers (including such commonly prescribed painkillers as morphine and oxycodone) are only minimally helpful for nerve pain.

Here are some other possible dangers that have been identified.

- Opioids can cause hyperalgesia (an intensifying of pain). They may create changes—perhaps even permanent changes—in the peripheral and central nervous systems and in your pain thresholds, possibly making you more sensitive to pain in the future.

- Opioids frequently have side effects. They can produce severe constipation, dry mouth, drowsiness, bladder problems, and even dangerous respiratory sedation. Many women also feel cognitively impaired on opioids. Sexual pain is bad enough without adding any of these conditions.

- Over time, opioids' ability to ease pain decreases, creating the risk of physical dependence. In medical terms, you develop "tolerance" for opioids, meaning that you have to take more and more of them

➤

> to get the same benefit you obtained at first. This can easily lead to physical dependence, requiring a withdrawal process that can be physically and psychologically devastating—and that should not be undertaken without a doctor's supervision.
>
> • Opioids are dangerous in excess or when mixed with other medications—and shouldn't be used at all if you drink alcohol or have liver or kidney problems.
>
> Obviously, you should work with your healthcare provider to manage all of these issues. If you are at the end of your rope and desperately need a break from your pain while your treatment is taking place, a course of opioid painkillers may be a reasonable temporary treatment, especially if your physician monitors you carefully and treats possible side effects (especially constipation) proactively, before they come up. Once again, you'll be walking a tightrope, balancing temporary pain relief with possible dangers. As always, listen to your instincts and work with a practitioner you trust.

ZEROING IN ON THE PROBLEM

Now that you understand something about the kind of chronic pain you may be experiencing, it's time to get more specific. We're going to help you figure out which disorders you may be suffering from, so that you can zero in on the Part 2 chapters that have helpful information about your possible condition.

Again, we're not encouraging you to do a self-diagnosis. You'll need to consult a knowledgeable physician to get a real diagnosis and to get treatment appropriate for your condition. But at least you can start to find out more about what you might have, and to gather research that you can share with your doctor.

Looking at the questionnaires that follow can be a stressful or even frightening experience, as you begin to focus on your symptoms and on the quality of your pain. As a former medical student, Deborah well remembers how anxious she and many of her classmates felt simply reading descriptions of diseases and lists of symptoms. Sooner or later, just about everyone in her class fell prey to "med student syndrome," in which every disease starts to sound like something you've got, and in which just the mention of a symptom triggers the sense that you are now suffering from that symptom too.

We urge you to get yourself in as calm a state as you can before completing these questionnaires. If you can, have a friend, a partner, or a family member with you while you fill them out—or if that idea doesn't suit you, at least make sure you have emotional support lined up for later if you need it.

Make sure to write down all your answers, and if you have any questions that arise from the process, write them down too. It's normal to feel anxious during a process like this one—but feeling anxious doesn't mean you can't get through it. You might turn to the relaxation exercises in Chapter 4 to help you get calm and to detach a bit from the process.

Okay, ready? Please complete the following questionnaires:

I. WHAT TYPE OF PAIN DO YOU HAVE?

For every question, please check all that apply.

A. What is the quality of your pain?

☐ burning

☐ itching/irritation

☐ throbbing

☐ aching

☑ stabbing *needling*

☐ sharp/shooting

☐ cramping

B. What is the nature of your pain?

☐ generalized

☑ localized

☐ radiating

☐ referred

☐ constant

☑ intermittent

☑ provoked

☐ unprovoked

C. If you checked "provoked," what kinds of stimuli might provoke your pain?

☑ sex

☐ physical contact

☐ wearing underwear

➤

□ exercise

□ anxiety

□ lack of sleep

□ sitting

□ walking

□ standing

□ stretching

D. Where is your pain located?

☑ clitoris

□ vestibule (vaginal opening)

□ vagina

□ labia

□ overall vulva

□ anus

□ groin

□ upper thighs

□ outer hips

□ lower back

E. What is the intensity of your pain? On a scale of 1 to 10, rate your pain (10 being the most painful).

_4_ now

_7_ on average for this week

_8_ at its worst this week

_2_ at its best this week

_8_ at its worst this month

II. WHAT KINDS OF SYMPTOMS DO YOU HAVE?

Circle the letter beside the cluster(s) of symptoms that describe your condition, even if you don't have every single symptom. (If in doubt, circle.)

A vulvar itching, burning, cracking, rawness, dryness, fragility, tenderness to the touch

B vaginal secretions that burn, aggravate, irritate, have abnormal odor

C exquisite tenderness to the touch or constant pain signals coming from the clitoris; a feeling of uncomfortable constant sexual arousal sometimes relieved with self-stimulation and orgasm; pain in the clitoris caused by sitting, certain leg movements, driving, tight clothing

D burning, stinging, itching, and/or throbbing as a result of touch at the vaginal opening; as touching or penetration continues, the area becomes numb in a peculiar way; burning pain specifically at urethral opening with touch or urination; after touch, a residual burning or itching may occur, lasting from minutes to days

E burning, irritation, and/or itchiness of a large area of the vulva without a dermatologic condition or visual appearance giving hints as to its cause (on either or both sides); a sudden sharp, lacerating, throbbing pain in the vaginal area, becoming worse when seated or touched, and mostly constant

➤

F extremely painful sensations of aching, burning, tightness, and muscle spasms in the genital area; right, left, or central pain at the vaginal opening or deeper in the vaginal canal with intercourse; crampy and throbby pain when provoked by touch; pain worsens as the day goes on and is worst at bedtime

G with penetration, a deep, sharp pain appears up in the vagina, usually on one side or the other but may be on both sides; stiffness in legs and hips in sexual positions; uncomfortable clicking in hip area or groin; radiation of sharp pain to the outer thigh, sometimes down to the knee, groin, or buttocks in certain positions

H intense bladder pain during vaginal intercourse; urgency to urinate during and after penetration; sexual touching causes pain flares; urinary frequency that may last days after sex; the constant feeling of needing to urinate even after just emptying; frequency of urination may disrupt sleep

I frequent pelvic/abdominal bloating that makes intimacy uncomfortable; gas pockets that hurt; residual pelvic discomfort after intercourse; anal pain with sex due to irritation or fissures

J pain with penetration that seems to be deep in the pelvis; severe cramps during period; backache; bladder pressure that is worse premenses and with menses; cyclic bloating and worsening of symptoms; pelvic tenderness after intercourse for hours or days

K heaviness and fullness in the pelvis; irregular or very heavy menstrual bleeding; deep pain with intercourse or penetration

L pelvic heaviness, on one or both sides, that increases as the day goes on; with intercourse or penetration, deep discomfort that may persist as residual pain for hours after; pelvic pain that is worse with menses

M sexual pain caused by touch; loss of elasticity after a surgical procedure, chemotherapy, or radiation therapy

N burning and tearing at the vaginal opening with touch, sometimes with small amounts of bleeding; discomfort in response to touch and/or tight clothing; a change in discharge to a thin, yellow, irritating type; stinging of urethra and surrounding skin during urination along with more frequent urination; weak pelvic floor muscles; feeling painfully tight in the muscles with intercourse

Key: Direct your attention to the chapters that explain your particular symptoms first. Remember though that you may have problems addressed in more than one chapter. The nerve pain and pelvic floor chapters are especially helpful to all to further understand painful sex.

A and B: Chapter 6	**F:** Chapter 10
C: Chapter 7	**G:** Chapter 11
D: Chapter 8	**H through L:** Chapter 12
E: Chapter 9	**M and N:** Chapter 13

As we discussed in Chapter 3, it will be helpful to bring the results of your questionnaires to your doctor for discussion.

SEEING THE PROBLEM IN LAYERS

Since so many of the women we treat have multiple conditions—and since the pelvis is such a complicated region—even if you're struggling with only one disorder, we've found it helpful to organize types of sexual pain into "layers," proceeding from the surface to the pelvis's deeper structures.

Of course, to some extent, this would be an oversimplification for any area of the body—and that is particularly true for the pelvis, which is in many ways the most "full" body area, containing many different organs and bodily functions. Every type of body tissue is in the pelvis (including skin, mucous membranes, muscles, nerves, ligaments, tendons, fascia, and bone), in addition to complicated organs (including the bowel, the bladder, and the reproductive system of the uterus, ovaries, and fallopian tubes).

Dysfunction in any of the above pelvic tissues or organs can result in painful sex. But we also have to give holistic attention to the rest of the body when figuring out why a woman has sexual pain. For instance, we have seen a severe connective tissue sprain in the shoulder pull on a woman's fascia all the way down into the hip and pelvic floor, causing her deep painful intercourse. Likewise, hormonal and inflammatory signals from elsewhere in the body may greatly affect the pelvis. And of course our brain, our most important sexual organ, responds to and regulates everything happening in our pelvis and sex lives.

Still, a little simplicity can be helpful in visualizing a complex medical condition. So here are the "layers" of the pelvis, so that you can identify which are the main ones giving you sexual pain.

The Surface Layer

The pelvic surface is the skin and mucous membrane (epidermis) of the vulva and of the pelvis in general. The skin itself is involved here, but so are all its appendages, including hair and sweat and oil glands. Also included are the mucous membranes, which include the surface of the vagina and its opening (the vestibule), as well as the openings of the urethra and anus. We explain pain in the surface layer of the pelvis in Chapters 6, 7, and 8.

The Nerve Layer

As we have seen, nerves travel throughout the pelvis, from deep within and out to its surface. In Chapter 9, we look at the peripheral nervous system, the central nervous system, and the autonomic nervous system, all of which help "run" the pelvis.

The Musculoskeletal Layer

The next deepest layer involves muscles, ligaments, tendons, fascia, and bones—the movement structures and support of the pelvis. These structures participate in virtually every type of sexual pain. We'll explore this layer in Chapters 10 and 11.

The Organ Layer

The fourth layer involves the deeper internal organs of the pelvis, including the bladder, which gives rise to a great deal of sexual pain. Endometriosis of the pelvic organs also causes deep sexual pain, and we'll talk about these conditions in Chapter 12.

The Systemic Layer

Finally, we have the bodywide layer of hormonal, immune, inflammatory, and surgical causes of sexual pain. You can read more about them in Chapter 13.

AN INTEGRATED APPROACH

Although we separate the pelvis into layers to better understand and visualize what's happening inside the body, in practice, we integrate the problems—and the solutions. Our twenty-two-year-old patient Sarah, for example, was frustrated by having seen so many physicians who could do little to help her with her deep aching and burning sexual pain. But when she came to us, we didn't try to treat her by ourselves. We brought in a physical therapist to help her, and we drew on specialists.

Sarah's treatment reflected our integrative philosophy. She began receiving specialized physical therapy to reduce her pelvic floor muscle spasms. She also started using several ointments for her various vulvar skin problems. She took an antihistamine to treat allergies contributing to the excess irritation in her vulvar skin. To calm her nerve pain, we prescribed the serotonin–norepinephrine reuptake inhibitor (SNRI) duloxetine (Cymbalta), an antidepressant that also treats centralized pain conditions such as fibromyalgia.

It wasn't easy treating Sarah, because she'd been suffering for five years before she came to us, and her damaged nerves insisted on transmitting one pain signal after another before we finally figured out how to make them stop. After six months, however, her multifaceted treatment was highly successful, and she went on to enjoy a pain-free life.

POTENTIAL BREAKTHROUGHS: LOOKING TOWARD THE FUTURE

Medical research on the biology of pain and its treatment is finally advancing in leaps and bounds, as chronic pain is now recognized as a major negative influence on the quality of life for all of us. For painful sex disorders, this research has been extremely helpful. For example, when Deborah was in medical school, the prevailing view was that damage to the nervous system was permanent and hopeless, and that nerves could never really heal. Since then, we have discovered how wrong this concept was, and more recent studies show the remarkable ability of even the brain (for example, in stroke victims) to rewire and find ways to compensate for damage. This knowledge informs us on sexual pain caused not only by nerve dysfunction, but also on all kinds of pelvic pain. Ongoing research gives us enormous optimism about curing your devastating type of pain, sexual pain.

6

SKIN AND
VAGINAL
PAIN

When people think of pain, they usually don't think of itching. But I think itching is the most torturous form of pain. With many forms of pain, you can take medication to at least take the edge off. With itching, there is little you can do to relieve it. And the more you scratch, the worse it gets. I literally thought I was going out of my mind.

I had never felt such intense itching in my life. I first used over-the-counter topical creams, and after a few days, when I saw no change, I finally went to see my gynecologist. He looked at me and said it didn't look like a yeast infection, but he prescribed an antifungal and he assured me that it would work.

It did not work, and when I called him back, he just prescribed stronger medications that also didn't work. I finally went to see another gynecologist, one recommended by a friend, and he had nothing useful to offer. He did do a vulva biopsy and said it showed nothing but inflammation. Not a big help.

I remember going into the bathroom at night, using scissors and a nail file to try to scratch the skin off—that is how bad the itching was. I know that sounds crazy, and when I talk about it, it sounds insane to me. But that is what such intense itching can do

*to a person. I remember at night praying to God to just stop this
suffering, because I didn't know how long I could last.*

—MARY, A TEACHER IN HER FORTIES

SKIN PAIN: AN OVERVIEW

Itching so intense that it is actually pain. Misdiagnosis of your condition as a
yeast infection, with treatment that only makes the problem worse. Dismissal
and disregard from the very doctors who are supposed to help you.

This is standard fare for any woman whose sexual pain arises from
dermatological conditions that cause painful skin breakage in the genital
area. If you're suffering from genital skin pain, you already know that the
resulting itching, burning, and sensitivity can make it unbearable to wear
jeans, let alone to tolerate sexual contact. And most gynecologists and der-
matologists are all too ignorant of the conditions that might be causing your
symptoms.

If you have a skin condition that is causing you sexual pain, you may
be wondering whether any medical treatment could even begin to help you.
Rest easy—there are many effective treatments, and you can almost certainly
find relief from pain and perhaps even a total healing of your condition. As
always, the first step is understanding, so read on to find out more.

HOW SKIN PAIN AFFECTS YOU

A chronic, painful skin condition makes sex less comfortable because the
surface seal of your skin is weakened. The top layer may actually shed when
your skin is touched (as happens with lichen sclerosus, covered later in this
chapter). Or perhaps your skin is ulcerated and the top layer is already off
(as happens with lichen planus, also covered later in this chapter). Sexual
contact will cause raw skin to itch and burn.

Another impediment to sex is the anticipation of residual pain: the days of pain that follow the "trauma" triggered by even comfortable sex—as the breaks, fissures, and cuts take time to heal, and the pain takes time to wane. If your genital skin is weak only on the outer labia, you might have an easier time with penetration or intercourse, but still, intimate touch may be difficult, since your skin may be so irritated that you don't want anyone to touch you. Lastly, pain in your genital area might decrease your libido.

SYMPTOMS OF SKIN CONDITIONS

If you have a skin-based problem with sexual pain, you are likely to have one or more of the following symptoms:

- a burning, itchy, irritated, fragile feeling;

- pain when involved area is touched;

- pain in various parts of the labia, clitoris, perineum, vestibule, and anal areas or generalized irritation of the vulva;

- contact bleeding from the delicate skin; and/or

- burning pain with urination when the urine touches the skin in passing.

WHAT'S GOING ON: THE BIOLOGY

Our skin is our largest organ. It divides and connects our inner and outer worlds, and it protects our inner world from the toxins and dangers that lurk outside. Powerful and vulnerable at the same time, this enormous organ responds to everything that happens on either side of the barrier, which is why stress of all kinds—emotional and physical—can cause flare-ups and irritations on our skin and mucous membranes, including the vulva and vagina.

In other words, skin is connected to everything and is involved in all of our functioning—and it is much more complicated than it looks!

Actually, we have two types of covering. Skin—which covers our public parts—has a relatively tough and impervious surface. Mucous membranes line our more intimate areas (mouths, lips, nostrils, eyelids, ears, genitals, anus, and other damp areas) and help keep them moist by secreting fluids.

The genital skin in particular is very involved in sexual activity. To function optimally, it needs to be strong, healthy, moist, and elastic. It covers and protects the vaginal opening and the sensitive clitoris. It contains the usual structures: hair, for protection; secretory glands, which release lubrication and pheromones (hormones involved in sexual arousal); and sweat glands, which help regulate body temperature by releasing perspiration. For many women, sexual pleasure is enhanced by touching the genital skin, so in a way, it's not "just" skin, it's more than that.

The skin covering our vulva and vagina can become irritated and painful in a variety of ways. Because the vulva "lives" in a dark, warm, and moist environment under our clothing, it is slightly more prone than other skin areas to become irritated. By the time we're in our midtwenties, virtually all of us have known some type of vulvar or vaginal irritation. Usually, these problems clear up on their own or in response to our physician's first line of treatment.

More serious conditions can cause painful skin breakage in the genital area, which creates itching, burning, scarring, and the possibility of infection. These conditions may resist treatment longer, especially if they are misdiagnosed and inappropriately treated. Chronic skin changes and vaginal imbalance can set in, making treatment a more difficult and lengthier process.

As we saw in Chapter 5, the longer you live with chronic pain, including painful itching, the greater the possibility of developing neuropathic pain, whereby your nerves keep sending "pain" or "itching" signals to your brain, even after the condition has cleared up. So our goal for sexual skin pain is always rapid and specific treatment.

Common Temporary Skin Conditions That May Cause Pain

There are several common types of skin pain, most of which are acute or minor. Although these can cause some irritation or discomfort in the genital area, they don't really interfere seriously or for long with sexual activity or pleasure. These types of disorders are also fairly easy to diagnose and treat, so if any of them is your primary problem, a competent gynecologist or dermatologist should be able to help you relatively quickly.

INFECTIOUS DISEASES

Many transient skin conditions are caused by bacteria, yeast, or viruses. However, these conditions shouldn't have any ongoing effect on your sexual activity.

CONTACT AND ALLERGIC REACTIONS

These are problems that develop when your skin or mucous membrane comes in contact with an irritating chemical or an allergen (something you're allergic to). Your genital skin can also respond to substances you inhale or eat, which can make this diagnosis a little more difficult. But usually, these conditions are easy to identify and treat. Be aware, though, that they can easily be confused with eczema or LSC, which we talk about in more detail below, under "Vulvar Conditions."

HORMONAL CAUSES OF SKIN CHANGE

Temporary vaginal inflammation and vulvar skin thinning and pain may be due to menopausal changes or other hormonal problems. These problems can cause sexual pain and can resemble other skin conditions, but they are treated very differently, so make sure your doctor doesn't confuse the diagnosis. If, along with your skin problems, you are having irregular menses or hot flashes, have been treated with estrogen-lowering medications such as leuprolide (Lupron Depot), have recently had a baby, or are struggling with thyroid or other hormonal issues, your problem probably doesn't stem from your skin itself, but from your hormones, so please see Chapter 13.

Cancerous and Precancerous Cells

Skin cancer in the genital area is rare, but genital skin cancer and precancer (usually of the squamous-cell type) do exist. Since localized pain with sex may be this cancer's first symptom, we always want to check for it if a woman reports pain during sex. Also, it is important to be aware that the frequency of cancer and precancer of the anal skin, and of the lowest part of the canal just inside the anus, is on the rise. Both vulvar and anal cancer are related to previous infection with human papillomavirus, especially in people with poor immune systems. Warning signs include an area of pain that doesn't heal, bumpiness, fragility, and skin that feels rough or bleeds to the touch. If you notice any such signs, your doctor should take a biopsy and have a pathologist analyze it for cancer cells. For anal opening and anal canal precancer and cancer, new screening techniques with anal Pap smears and high-resolution anoscopy (HRA) (the use of a magnifying scope to see and biopsy early tiny precancers in the anal canal) are now available. Anal and vulvar cancer detected early is curable. If you do develop this cancer, you'll need surgery to remove the cancerous lesion, followed by other treatments such as chemotherapy and radiation.

Inflammation and Chronic Skin Conditions

Most of the chronic skin conditions that cause sexual pain have a basis that's different from the ones we just saw. Although a lot remains to be learned about these disorders, chronic skin conditions seem to be caused by some combination of autoimmune reactions and chronic inflammation.

These conditions are interrelated. Inflammation is a set of side effects produced by our immune reactions—the chemical cascade released as the body tries to fight off what it perceives as a threat to the system. Autoimmune and allergic reactions are directed to a type of "false threat," as the body overreacts to an otherwise benign substance, such as some type of food, or perhaps a chemical or cell of the body itself. In a way that we don't yet fully understand, the inflammation and resulting problems may continue even when the initial trigger is no longer present, as the system keeps flooding itself with immune chemicals, which can in turn cause other dangerous side effects. Stressors of various kinds (an illness or a physical strain, insufficient rest or nutrition, or emotional stress) seem to make things worse, causing flare-ups or prolonging the condition.

While we don't know all we'd like to know about the causes of chronic skin pain, we're learning more every day, with hopeful possibilities for improved understanding and better treatments. Meanwhile, one thing is clear: The better care you take of yourself—physically, mentally, and emotionally— the more resources you will have to combat chronic skin and sexual pain.

Kinds of Skin Disorders

Disorders in the genital area fall into two categories, general and vulvar/ vaginal. General skin conditions can take place anywhere on our body's surface but are particularly uncomfortable on the vulva. Vulvar/vaginal conditions tend to occur mainly or only in that particular area (see illustration 6-1 for diagram of the vulva).

GENERAL SKIN DISORDERS

The general conditions are far easier to diagnose and to treat. Since they also occur in men and children, and in other body parts, they are better recognized by physicians and have more available treatment options.

Treatments usually consist of some combination of topical and oral medications. You can generally expect your treatment to last about two weeks and to produce permanent, lasting results. Some conditions though, including psoriasis and eczema, are permanent: They can usually be treated and put into very good remission, but the possibility of future flare-ups exists.

The following are general conditions that may cause sexual pain, but usually only in a mild or transient way. If you think you may have one of

Illustration 6-1.

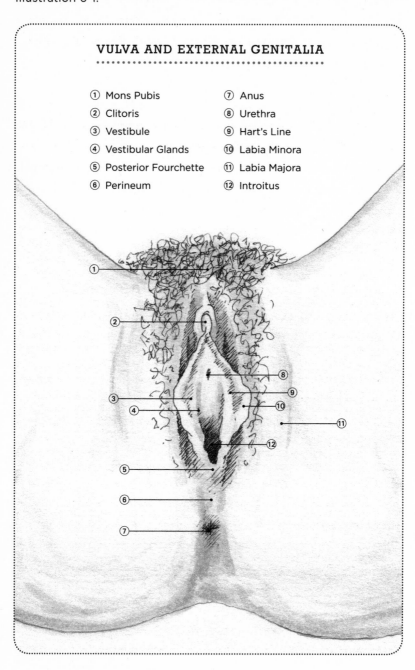

VULVA AND EXTERNAL GENITALIA

1. Mons Pubis
2. Clitoris
3. Vestibule
4. Vestibular Glands
5. Posterior Fourchette
6. Perineum
7. Anus
8. Urethra
9. Hart's Line
10. Labia Minora
11. Labia Majora
12. Introitus

these disorders, talk to your physician, but rest assured that these conditions are treatable and are only temporary. Unless they are ignored for a very long time, they should not become chronic, nor should they cause significant sexual pain.

Eczema

This is an itchy, irritated rash that's red, dry, and often cracked and leathery. It appears most commonly on the scalp, face, neck, elbows, knees, and buttocks, but it can appear on the vulva as well. It's allergy-based, springing ultimately from genetic, immune-system, and/or environmental causes, and it tends to flare up with stress.

Psoriasis

You can identify this condition by its thick silvery scales and itchy, dry, red patches, which are sometimes painful. Psoriasis is a common chronic auto-immune skin disease that affects the life cycle of skin cells, causing them to build up rapidly on the skin's surface.

Vitiligo

In this condition, white, depigmented skin patches occur throughout the body. When vitiligo appears on the vulva, the patches tend to be delicate and more easily irritated than the surrounding skin.

Hair-Follicle Infections

You would notice these as irritations and bumps or pimples at the places of the vulva that are laden with hair. Each individual hair follicle may feel like a bump. Shaving or waxing may be a trigger. Research shows that an allergy to a fungus that dwells deep in the hair follicle may be involved.

Sebaceous and Other Skin Cysts

These also feel like tender bumps or pimples. They can be found at the sebaceous glands in the labia, which become clogged by rubbing or from a microtrauma (a bump or bruise too small to cause dramatic damage but that nevertheless can be painful or irritating).

Bacterial and Fungal Infections

These appear as persistent red rashes on the vulvar skin. As we've seen, they are often confused with the more serious chronic disorders.

Viral Infections

Intimate contact can transmit a number of viral infections, including herpes (characterized by painful blisters in the genital area) and molluscum contagiosum (characterized by similar, but painless bumps).

Another recently recognized vulvar condition of painful, large, but transient blisters is caused by the Epstein-Barr virus—the same virus that causes mononucleosis. As you might guess, this disturbing condition often occurs in teens. Blood antibody testing for Epstein-Barr is useful for diagnosis. In rare cases, this type of blistering can recur again and again, in which case the culprit may be an autoimmune condition called Behçet's disease, for which ongoing specialty care is needed.

Extreme Drying

Sometimes overcleaning and overwiping can irritate the genital area. This condition is surprisingly common—and is easily fixed by a change in hygiene habits. Many women overclean the anal area after a bowel movement, leading to sometimes severe chronic cracking and skin fissures that extend up over the perineum to the vaginal opening, causing painful sex. Instead we advise taking a quick shower rinse or using a squirt bottle to remove stool at the anal opening, and then pat dry with a soft cotton cloth. If you are out of the house, use just one gentle wipe with a hypoallergenic baby wipe to clean, and then air dry. Following up with a coating of natural oil, such as vitamin E, to the anal opening will allow this area to heal.

Contact Dermatitis, Allergic Reactions, and Drug Reactions

If you've been in direct contact with an irritating chemical, if you've eaten or inhaled an allergen, or if you take a medication you're allergic to, you might develop a tender, itchy, red rash, sometimes with a feeling like hives. Try to figure out what set off the reaction. The most common allergens affecting the vulva are fragrances in toiletries and cosmetics.

Warts (Condylomata)

These bumps are painless unless infected or injured. In the genital area, they're acquired by intimate contact. A number of good treatment options are available. However, please note that any wart that looks unusual or does not respond to treatment does need to be biopsied to evaluate for precancer and cancer of the vulvar or anal skin.

MAINLY VULVAR DISORDERS

In contrast to the general conditions, the mainly vulvar disorders are more complex and even mysterious—and, until recently, underresearched. As we just saw, skin disorders that primarily occur on the vulva seem to be caused by a malfunction of the skin's immune and inflammatory functions. As a result, the protective seal of the skin and mucous membrane is compromised, and it may be weakened, broken, raw, or marked by abrasions and breaks.

These conditions are much harder to diagnose. To identify them properly, your physician must look at your skin with magnification, which many doctors fail to do. As a result, vulvar disorders are often confused with the more general skin conditions. If a doctor treats you for the wrong disorder, your own disorder lingers and becomes far harder to treat, so the stakes for finding a good doctor are high. Be aware, though, that you might have one of these more complex, systemic conditions *and* a more general or superficial condition, such as a yeast infection, eczema, or psoriasis. Your physician will need to look deeper and treat both the minor condition and the major one.

Because these chronic inflammatory conditions are such major causes of sexual pain, we'll look at them in detail in the next section.

CHRONIC SKIN CONDITIONS: THE SPECIFICS

Now let's talk specifics: the most common skin disorders causing chronic sexual pain. We're focusing only on chronic pain, because the acute vaginal infections that cause skin and sexual pain are far more easily recognized by most doctors and are also easier to treat.

WHAT IS LICHEN?

Lichen is short for lichenification, which is thickening of the skin and prominence of skin markings due to chronic rubbing or scratching (the itch–scratch cycle). It is often superimposed upon another dermatologic disorder, such as psoriasis, eczema, lichen sclerosus—anything that itches.

VULVAR CONDITIONS

These occur primarily on the vulva and are the main culprits causing sexual pain. Here they are in approximate order of most to least common.

Lichen Simplex Chronicus (LSC)

This condition is closely related to eczema, and, like eczema, it appears to be caused by a combination of autoimmune conditions and inflammation. However, its appearance on the vulva is usually somewhat different: it creates an itchy, burning feeling, as well as red and whitish skin changes, with cracking, and it also makes more prominent the skin's normal small wrinkles, folds, and bumps in a butterfly-like pattern around the labia.

LSC occurs in women of all ages, and it appears most often in those who have a history of allergies. Biopsies of women with LSC reveal surface thickening and inflammatory cells in skin layers, suggesting that it is a condition sparked by inflammation. Sexual friction or sexual activity generally may be very painful and may cause burning and itching of the skin, both while it's being touched and afterward.

Chronic Vulvovaginal Candidiasis

Although this condition can masquerade as LSC, it often includes more tissue swelling, redness, and cracking. It is caused by fungal (usually *Candida albicans*) infections of the skin and vaginal canal, making it a potentially acute and easily treatable condition.

However, this is one of those conditions in which diagnosis is often simply missed, and if the disease goes untreated long enough, it may become chronic. It takes up to two weeks to clear the skin of the fungal forms, so sometimes, even if treatment is given, it isn't used long enough. If a resistant type of fungus is present, the usual treatment won't work, and again, the condition might become chronic. Systemic problems such as diabetes may also cause yeast infections to become chronic.

Even though treatment of a chronic condition is harder, we do have good success treating this form of chronic fungal infection when the correct diagnosis is finally made. As with LSC, sexual friction or sexual activity generally may be very painful, due to the preexisting irritation, which may burn and cause great itching of the skin—both while it's being touched and afterward.

Seborrheic Vulvitis

In this condition, hair follicles and sebaceous (oil) glands are inflamed, producing irritation and itching of the vulvar skin. This condition often appears similar to LSC, but when skin is viewed with magnification, the inflammation at the hair follicles becomes evident. The sexual symptoms, however, are similar to those of LSC and candidiasis.

Chronic Bartholin's or Skene's Cysts

You have two sets of glands near the vaginal opening—Bartholin's and Skene's—both of which can develop cysts or abscesses. Fortunately, the cysts are usually well recognized and easy to treat with injections, drainage, or excision. Until they have healed (which takes about two weeks), they can affect your sex life by causing pain during penetration, as their swelling blocks the vaginal opening.

Recurrent or Recalcitrant Genital Herpes Flares

Genital herpes is a chronic viral disease that creates blisters, then ulcers, in the genital area, producing moderate to severe burning pain that may get much worse with sex. Outbreaks last for about a week, and come and go—making herpes difficult to diagnose, since you need to identify and culture the blister at the time you are in pain. It is often hard to schedule your doctor's exam to coincide with the pain flare, but it's important, so please try to do so. Of course, you would prefer the herpes to be "silent," since less-active herpes is less likely to cause chronic sexual pain. Antiviral medications are extremely effective in quieting this chronic infection.

Lichen Sclerosus (LS)

This condition can occur on any part of the body, but usually, we find it on the vulva. It appears as a "cigarette paper" patch of vulvar skin, either localized (a single patch) or widespread (much or most of the vulva). LS thins the tissues and decreases elasticity to such an extent that the tissues often tear easily with intimate touch, which creates great pain for any type of sexual activity. As LS progresses, it often obliterates the usual vulvar architecture (including causing adhesions over the clitoris), making arousal and orgasm difficult or impossible. It also may shrink the labia minora and the mucous membranes at the vaginal opening, making penetration almost impossible. Meanwhile, the vulvar skin continues to erode, so that it cracks easily with intimate sexual contact.

LS is believed to be an autoimmune condition, as the body's inflammatory cells attack the surface layers of skin. Biopsies show severe thinning of the skin layers. The condition can be found among people of all ages, but it's most common in children and in women over age fifty, where it occurs in up to 1 woman in 60. If you're going through menopause, don't assume your sexual pain is the natural result of getting older: You may simply need to be treated for LS. Long-term follow-up with your doctor is necessary, because studies show that women with LS have a 6 percent chance of developing vulvar cancer.

Hidradenitis Suppurativa

Pus-filled nodules interconnect deep under the vulvar skin in this rare, chronic, recurrent, and severely painful autoimmune condition. Due to the infections that can occur, this is one of the most debilitating types of skin pain, and the resulting skin tracks and scars lead to yet more infection. When you have this condition, you feel very uncomfortable at any genital touch, and the infected nodules can actually become worse and spread with sexual pressure. Surgical treatment is best for moderate and severe cases.

Lichen Planus (LP)

Fortunately this most painful of all vulvar disorders is one of the least common. It takes the form of painful, burning, itching red lesions and violet, flat papules (small, solid, rounded bumps). These tend to ulcerate, becoming sharply demarcated erosions of different sizes, often in the vestibule, negating any possibility of intercourse. The condition is associated with faint white lines in the vulvar skin, called Wickham striae, which aid in diagnosis. LP is an autoimmune disease that can also occur in the mouth and vaginal canal. It strikes primarily middle-aged and older women—the median age is fifty-five. LP can be extremely hard to diagnose and sometimes doesn't show up clearly in a biopsy, meaning that physicians must rely on the impressions they form during a careful magnified vulvar-skin examination.

VAGINAL CONDITIONS

These are often caused by an imbalanced or altered vaginal flora (here, "flora" means "bacterial environment"). They can cause discomfort with sex due to the associated vaginal discharge, which often irritates the vaginal opening (that is, the vestibule) and vulvar skin. See illustration 6-1 to note the

COMMON MISDIAGNOSES FOR
CHRONIC SKIN AND VAGINAL DISORDERS

MISDIAGNOSIS	HOW TO RULE IT OUT
Recurrent yeast infection	Wet smear, specific fungal culture, or DNA test
Bacterial vaginosis	Wet smear, pH measurement, bacterial culture
Recurrent bladder infection	Specific urine analysis and bacterial cultures
Menopausal "atrophy"	Appearance, wet smear, cultures, symptoms
Genital warts	Magnified exam of skin, possible biopsy
Overactive bladder syndrome	Symptoms persist after treatment
Psychological illness	MD awareness/education

limits of the vagina (within the opening), the vestibule, and the vulvar skin itself, which is only located outward from Hart's line in the vaginal opening.

The most common vaginal disorder that causes sexual pain is called desquamative inflammatory vaginitis (DIV). This somewhat mysterious vaginal-lining disorder is partly an autoimmune condition. It might coexist with another autoimmune condition, lichen planus (covered on the previous page). Sexual pain caused by DIV takes the form of burning at the vaginal opening, making touch and vaginal penetration painful, and intercourse also increases the profuse, irritating, yellow discharge.

We don't know what triggers DIV. In about half the cases Deborah has treated, she has seen the condition develop after antibiotic use or diarrheal illness, but the triggers for the other half of her DIV patients remain mysterious. The underlying cause of the illness involves a shift in vaginal homeostasis: The lactobacilli (a type of bacteria) that keep the vaginal environment stable seem to have been destroyed, creating a less acidic environment. Shedding of the cells lining the vaginal canal is another feature, thinning the inner vagina and making intercourse very painful.

This painful condition can definitely be treated, but ongoing maintenance may be necessary. Local anti-inflammatories, estrogen, and oral antibiotics are helpful, as is treatment with probiotics.

DIAGNOSIS: THE TESTS YOU NEED

Chronic sexual pain is one of the most commonly misdiagnosed and mistreated conditions in all of medicine. We've seen dozens of patients whose doctors didn't perform the correct diagnostic tests to properly identify their disorders—or, in some cases, didn't perform any tests at all but instead simply relied on a quick look. This section is to help you ensure that your physician is ordering the right tests to create an accurate diagnosis and treatment plan. If he or she is not ordering these tests, you probably want to consider finding another doctor.

Vulvar Skin Conditions

The essential first step here is a good vulvar skin exam using magnification, since to the naked eye, many skin conditions look similar to each other. Even with magnification, the different types of lichens may be difficult to distinguish, so you may also need a small skin biopsy.

Your physician must send the skin biopsy to a lab pathologist with dermatologic expertise—not just expertise in gynecology. It's easy to make a mistake with skin conditions, which is why special stains for fungi or viruses may also be necessary. If the results of the biopsy don't accord well with your condition's physical appearance, your physician may consult a dermatologic specialist. Sometimes the biopsy result may not give a specific diagnosis, and your doctor may need to rely on his or her visual impression to decide on a treatment. Then responses to your treatment (whether good or poor) may be very helpful in determining your diagnosis and ultimate treatment.

Other tests may include:

- cultures for bacteria, fungi, and viruses, to rule out a coexisting infection;

- a wet smear of vaginal secretions;

- certain blood tests to further evaluate inflammatory or autoimmune conditions—for example, LS often coexists with autoimmune thyroid abnormalities;

- blood allergy testing or patch testing to rule out an allergic or contact irritant.

Vaginal Conditions

It is *essential* that your doctor perform a speculum exam to evaluate the appearance of the mucous membrane of the vaginal canal and any secretions on the inside vaginal wall.

The next step is a microscopic evaluation with a saline wet prep slide to evaluate the cells of the inner vaginal wall and any secretions present. A swab is used to pick up some secretions from your vagina, and using a pH paper, a measurement of the acid/alkaline balance is made. This is useful in differentiating different types of vaginal conditions. Secretions are also mixed with saline on a microscope slide (called a "wet smear") to view the state of the vaginal cells and the vaginal environment, analyzing lining cells, immune cells, bacteria, and fungi. Then, potassium hydroxide is added to the slide to "dissolve" out the many vaginal lining cells so that the fungi and bacteria in between them are more easily seen. In difficult cases, a Gram stain may be done, in which a microscope slide of the vaginal secretions is dyed to help diagnose in more detail which exact bacteria are present.

TRYING TO STAY MOTIVATED

Savannah had spent her professional life counseling other women to care for their bodies and their reproductive health. When she had to care for her own sexual pain, however, she encountered roadblocks she'd never expected.

"I've been a sexual person my whole life, but [with sexual pain,] everything about your body becomes so medicalized," she says. "Sometimes I am not compliant with the things I have to do, because it's always a reminder of what is wrong with me. I have to use about four hundred million creams! Sometimes I am very proactive and want to take control over my health, for both me and my partner's sake, but there are other times when I just don't want to deal with it."

Although Savannah sometimes finds using her creams cumbersome, thankfully these are safe and effective medications, and when used regularly, they keep her symptoms at bay. The regular use of these creams just became part of her normal routine, like shaving her legs or tweezing her eyebrows—she may not always like it, but she knows doing it will make her feel better about herself.

TREATMENTS: WHAT YOU CAN EXPECT

If you get the proper treatment, there's no reason to think you can't get better, function well sexually, and avoid recurring flare-ups of sexual pain. Your skin may always be sensitive, but even if a flare-up does occur, resuming the treatment usually produces another remission. The key is to get the proper diagnosis right at the beginning, so you can get the proper treatment. Meanwhile, follow the genital wellness suggestions in Chapter 4.

For Vulvar Conditions

The mainstay of treatment for painful chronic vulvar skin conditions is topical anti-inflammatory medications. These are quite effective and can bring relief within two to four weeks, with the prospect of healing the skin completely within eight to twelve weeks, depending on how long the condition has been going on and whether inappropriate (and irritating) medication has been previously applied. Even if your condition can't be completely cured, you can look forward to lengthy periods of remission, or even permanent remission.

LSC, LS, and LP can be effectively treated with corticosteroids in the form of ointments. Avoid creams though, since they contain irritants. Your doctor will have you apply this treatment directly to the skin in well-controlled doses and for limited periods of time. In some cases, you can eventually switch to a more natural skin protectant to keep the condition controlled. Continue to have your skin checked at regular three- to six-month intervals, and be prepared for an occasional repeat course of medication for flare-ups.

Sometimes LP is treated with corticosteroid suppositories applied to the vaginal entrance. If this treatment isn't effective, you might try topical immune modulators, such as tacrolimus (Protopic) and pimecrolimus (Elidel), which decrease your body's autoimmune activity. Your physician will probably also prescribe topical hormone creams and anesthetic ointments, such as lidocaine, for pain. Sometimes antifungal medications are also necessary, as well as antifungal shampoo to wash the area twice a week. Although we try to avoid them (due to the fact that they often cause fungal overgrowth), antibiotics are occasionally needed to treat bacterial infection in areas of fissuring and ulcerations. In the most difficult cases, your physician may administer corticosteroid or hormonal injections directly into the painful tissues.

Meanwhile, your topical treatments may be supplemented with oral medications, particularly antihistamines to calm the itching and irritation and to lower the activity of the mast cells in the inflamed tissues. Montelukast

(Singulair) can also prevent the local immune chemicals in your skin from causing irritation. In the most difficult cases, your doctor might prescribe oral corticosteroids or medications to calm the reactions of your nervous system to the pain, such as amitriptyline (Elavil).

You should strongly consider physical therapy as part of your treatment, since soft-tissue mobilization—massage of the connective tissue just under the skin's surface—helps prevent scarring and thickening. Physical therapy also gets the blood flowing, which is needed for healing, and it also corrects the pelvic floor muscle-gripping and spasms that are a common reflex response to the skin pain (see the "Physical Therapy" section in Chapter 10 for more details).

Occasionally, surgery is necessary to treat adhesions that may have developed as a result of LS or LP. Generally, procedures focus on the area around the clitoris and labia, but surgery may also be used to widen the vaginal opening if it has become scarred from inflammation.

If none of these treatments work, LSC and eczema might occasionally be treated with special light therapy in courses of treatment every two to three weeks for two to three months. Other treatments for LP and LS include the newer biologicals—antibodies that modulate the immune system to correct autoimmune triggers.

In all cases, keeping the area strong and elastic is a main treatment goal.

For Vaginal Conditions

As with vulvar conditions, topical agents are best and are central to treatment. Their focus in this case is to restore the normal flora of the vagina, correcting the bacterial environment and allowing new growth to replace the eroded cells of the vaginal lining. Estriol gelcaps can help strengthen the vaginal layers; probiotics will help restore the "good bacteria"; and boric acid suppositories and antifungals can help protect against fungal infection. These treatments have all been proven helpful—both short term, and as maintenance once or twice a week over the long term. In some cases, you'll also need topical antibiotics, such as clindamycin and metronidazole. Topical medications may be supplemented with oral medications—primarily anti-fungals but sometimes antibiotics or short courses of anti-inflammatories.

HOW *NOT* TO TREAT SKIN-RELATED SEXUAL PAIN

Do *not* . . .

- ignore diarrhea that may be irritating the vulvar skin.

- apply any substance if you haven't read the list of ingredients.

- apply anything that contains propylene glycol, benzocaine, parabens, or other chemicals. If you have not heard of a listed additive, cannot pronounce it, or cannot read it because it is in a foreign language, chances are high it is not good for your genital skin! And products made in China often have unlisted toxic ingredients. The simpler the product the better.

- apply topical steroids without first consulting a physician.

- apply antifungal topical treatments unless your physician has specifically tested for and found a yeast infection (if you don't have one, antifungals can make things worse).

- take any type of antibiotic, whether oral or topical, without consulting a physician (it could worsen your condition, cause painful side effects, and make you resistant to antibiotics, making treatment of future infections difficult).

›

> - resort to laser treatments—research has shown them to be inadequate.

> - allow your physician to perform surgical excision of skin lesions until he or she has tried less-severe treatments (often, less-invasive treatments work, if given time).

> - ignore coexisting conditions that also need treatment—if you have developed additional disorders, you won't fully recover until they are also treated.

POTENTIAL BREAKTHROUGHS: LOOKING TOWARD THE FUTURE

According to vulvar dermatologist Grace Bandow, MD, the cooperation between dermatology and gynecology is growing rapidly. "I think the field is becoming better established with the International Society for the Study of Vulvovaginal Disease and through their meetings and website," she says. "The more coordinated we become nationally and internationally, the better we can manage rarer diseases like lichen planus, which are nearly impossible to study without a multicenter approach."

Dr. Bandow also sees hopeful research developments on the horizon. "Probably the most exciting advancement in dermatology in the last ten to fifteen years is the class of drugs called biologic agents [the antibodies we mentioned above]." She says, "Approved for psoriasis and psoriatic arthritis, among other rheumatologic conditions, off-label use of these agents for rarer diseases like lichen planus has sometimes been very successful."

Savannah and Mary were able to get the treatment they needed, and although both are facing a long, slow road to recovery, each feels ultimately hopeful. "I have my bad days, and I have my good days, but I know things are moving in the right direction," Mary says. Savannah is still struggling with her "loss of innocence"—her realization, at age thirty-one, that she can't take her own body and her sexuality for granted, as she always thought she could. But she and her partner continue to enjoy each other sexually, and she is looking forward to reclaiming her libido and her sexual self now that most of her condition has cleared up.

If you are struggling with a skin condition, we want to assure you that your pain can be treated. But to ensure that your nerves and muscles don't get involved, time is of the essence, so if you haven't yet found the right physician, please keep looking (and see Chapter 3).

This is an area where a great deal of research offers us new reasons for hope every day. Better topical and oral medications are continually being developed, and new discoveries about chronic inflammation and autoimmune disorders will also help enormously. Environmental improvements will help lessen the toxin exposure for all of us, and new genetic studies are also shedding light on the problem. We are also hopeful about the way that physicians are generally getting much better at recognizing the need to address coexistent disorders and to treat skin problems in conjunction with other conditions that make them worse. All in all, there are many reasons for hope, on both a personal and a medical level, and if your painful sex is a result of skin problems, you will get better.

7

CLITORAL PAIN

I was sitting in a meeting and I remember feeling like my clitoris was on fire. And I was practically in tears and was terrified and was trying to keep it together in a room full of men. The clitoris doesn't usually feel pain, and it's a very sensitive part of your genitals, and I was so frightened. This just completely freaked me out, and I didn't know what to do. At that point, I just hoped something had scratched me and the pain would go away.

—JESSIE, EARLY THIRTIES, BUSINESS EXECUTIVE

CLITORAL PAIN: AN OVERVIEW

Pain in the clitoris, or clitorodynia, is probably one of the most severe and emotionally disruptive types of sexual pain there is. It is also less common than other types of sexual pain, but that fact is of no comfort if you are one of the tens of thousands of women suffering from it. In fact, because of the silence and shame that typically surround this condition, you may feel even more isolated than you are—this is a topic that most women avoid speaking about, even to their physicians and therapists, and even when clitoral pain is the reason for the appointment.

Because of the silence surrounding this condition—both among women and in the medical community—we don't have any reliable statistics about it. But we have noticed (and our fellow clinicians confirm this impression) that more and more women seem to be reporting this type of pain. Perhaps, at long last, the silence is starting to break.

SYMPTOMS OF CLITORAL CONDITIONS

If you are suffering from pain in your clitoris, you are likely to have at least some of the following symptoms:

- exquisite tenderness from touch, or constant pain signals coming from the clitoris;

- a feeling of uncomfortable constant or intermittent swelling or sexual arousal, sometimes relieved by self-stimulation and orgasm;

- pain in the clitoris caused by sitting, certain leg movements, driving, or tight clothing; or

- after touch or orgasm, burning pain that sometimes lasts for hours or days.

Those of us who lived in the 1960s remember what a big deal it was when women began speaking frankly about the clitoris and its role in sexual pleasure. A new women's health movement was at least partly inspired by women seeking to move past "the myth of the vaginal orgasm" and to recognize how central the clitoris is in most women's sexual climax. Women began to celebrate this supremely sensitive part of their bodies, and many women still cheer when, at performances of Eve Ensler's play *The Vagina Monologues,* one of the characters points out that the clitoris has twice as many nerve endings as the penis, and can therefore presumably provide women with extra helpings of pleasure.

So what happens when what should be a source of joy becomes a source of pain?

Because the clitoris is perhaps the most sensitive part of your body, any pain there is amplified enormously. Shame, secrecy, and depression are aspects of most types of sexual pain—but never more so than when a woman's pain is located at the very center of her sexuality.

HOW CLITORAL PAIN AFFECTS YOU

While you have clitoral pain, you might feel the condition has taken over your life. Rest assured that treatments are available, and they offer excellent prospects for long-term freedom from pain. But while you're waiting for the treatments to work, you'll need plenty of patience, fortitude, and support.

Even after the pain is gone, many women feel anxious about sex for weeks or months afterward, making it difficult for them to reacquaint themselves with their own sexuality. Sexual pleasure is difficult to imagine when the slightest touch on the clitoris has once caused such pain.

"After I was treated, I was still terrified to have intercourse for the first few months," Jessie says. "I didn't know if intercourse would bring back the pain or make it spread. But now my husband and I are able to have intercourse with little anxiety."

Even when sex isn't involved, clitoral pain can play havoc with your life. Jessie told us that when her pain was at its worst, she hurt all the time, no matter what she was doing. She couldn't find a comfortable seated position, and she couldn't even wear underwear.

"The pain covers the clitoris, labia, and the very top part, where the pubic bone is," she says. "It hates any kind of light irritating touch (like underwear). It doesn't particularly like a rough touch, but a light touch is much more irritating, and sets the pain off like a fire alarm," she says.

"What makes my pain worse is wearing tight clothes, sitting—sitting in cars especially—and certain exercises, like the treadmill and elliptical," she says. "Also, not getting enough sleep makes my pain worse, because sleep is necessary to let my pelvic floor muscles rest."

Over and above the physical accommodations, Jessie frequently feels both depressed and anxious. "At the beginning, I was having massive panic attacks and was desperate and hopeless," she says. "I still go through phases of hopelessness. It affects my life all day, and pretty much every day. One of the most difficult emotions I have is envy that so many other people don't have to live like this. To quote my five-year-old, 'It's just not fair.'"

WHAT'S GOING ON: THE BIOLOGY

Because the clitoris plays a major role in female arousal and orgasm, it is well endowed with nerve endings, making this tiny area highly sensitive to touch, pressure, temperature, vibration, and chemicals. The primary nerve connecting the clitoris to the central nervous system is the pudendal nerve, but fibers from a host of other nerves heighten the sensitivity still further, including the upper pelvic nerves—the ilioinguinal, iliohypogastric, and genitofemoral nerves (see illustration 7-1 for the location of some of these nerves). In addition, through our system of connective tissue, and the round ligament, the clitoris is connected to the uterus and the other organs up in the pelvis. With the use of Magnetic Resonance Imaging (MRI), we are learning more and more about the complex anatomical details of this relatively unstudied organ, and how it enlarges and responds in sexual arousal.

The clitoris has its own muscles, which are connected to the pubic bone and to the other large muscles of the pelvic floor. Within the superficial layers of muscles at the vaginal opening (see illustration 10-2 in Chapter 10), and key to sexual arousal and orgasm, is a plexus (interwoven network) of blood vessels, which become engorged and enlarged as a result of sexual stimulation, and deflate and return to normal size after orgasm. So the clitoris is actually composed of several active structures under the skin and hidden from view, which wrap around the urethra and lower vagina and surround the vaginal opening, as seen in illustration 7-1. Two large erectile chambers,

Illustration 7-1.

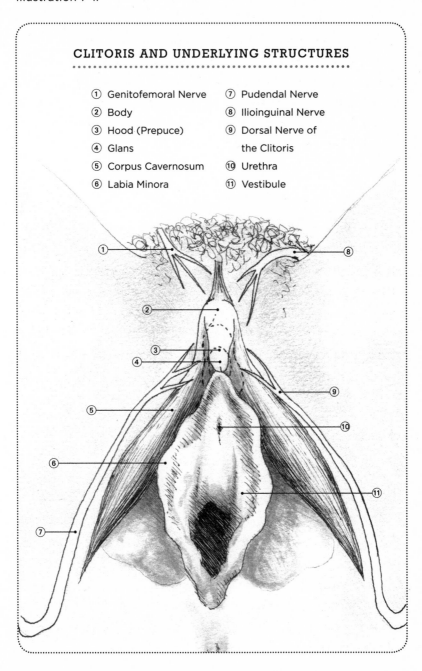

CLITORIS AND UNDERLYING STRUCTURES

① Genitofemoral Nerve   ⑦ Pudendal Nerve

② Body   ⑧ Ilioinguinal Nerve

③ Hood (Prepuce)   ⑨ Dorsal Nerve of

④ Glans   the Clitoris

⑤ Corpus Cavernosum   ⑩ Urethra

⑥ Labia Minora   ⑪ Vestibule

which underlie the labia and vestibule on each side, are called the corpora cavernosa, and hidden spongy elastic structures around the urethra and oval bulbs of tissue under the vestibule are together called the corpus spongiosum. The portions of the clitoris surrounding the urethra and extending under the lower vagina correspond to the Grafenberg spot (popularly known as the G-spot), which contributes to arousal and orgasm with vaginal penetration. These components all add up to form a complex functional whole organ that's up to six inches long, almost as large as the penis, and much more than the tiny "button" long thought to be the clitoris.

The extraordinary sensitivity, connectedness, size, and complexity of these structures mean that clitoral pain can be excruciating. Pain may be momentarily provoked by something as casual as a touch or a pair of panties, or it may be continuous, radiating, and unremitting. For a variety of reasons, the nerves in this sensitive organ can become irritated, leading to inappropriate random engorgement and muscle tension. For many women, along with the pain, comes an uncomfortable feeling of being aroused— which is made all the more disturbing if actually touching the clitoris, in an effort to relieve the arousal, is too painful.

Clitorodynia isn't the name of a specific disease—the suffix "odynia" simply means "pain." That pain can have a variety of causes, and a woman might be suffering from one, two, or several of the following:

- an overgrowth or extreme sensitization of the nerve fibers in or around the clitoris;

- recurrent herpes simplex or postherpetic neuralgia (a nerve disorder that can develop after a herpes infection);

- skin conditions (especially lichen sclerosus) that may be hidden under the clitoral hood, or chronic skin yeast infections, which can also be hidden under the clitoral hood or deep within a skin fold (see Chapter 6);

- spasms or tension in the pelvic floor muscles that surround the pudendal nerve's clitoral branch, which supplies most clitoral sensation (see Chapter 10);

- compression anywhere along the long pathway of the pudendal nerve, which has fibers that supply the clitoris (read all about the pudendal nerve in Chapter 9);

- the referral of pain downward, toward the clitoris, by the ilio-inguinal, iliohypogastric, or genitofemoral nerves, which might be irritated anywhere along their paths from the upper lumbar spine (see Chapter 9); scars from a cesarean section might create this problem;

- inappropriate filling of the erectile tissues with blood from an abnormal vessel, such as a varicose vein or an arteriovenous malformation;

- a blockage of blood vessels to the area (especially in the puden-dal artery), which decreases blood supply to the clitoral nerves;

- hip disorders that cause groin pain radiating to the clitoris (see Chapter 11);

- a small anatomical problem such as a cyst or neuroma (a small localized nerve tumor); or

- a side effect of medication, especially antidepressants such as trazodone and duloxetine (Cymbalta), which increase the brain's dopamine levels.

In addition to the above-listed side effects from medication and the nerve and blood-vessel problems, a chemical imbalance in the brain marked by high dopamine levels can lead to a distressing and painful condition called Persistent Genital Arousal Disorder (PGAD), in which a woman feels perpetually aroused. (See the boxed text.)

PERSISTENT GENITAL AROUSAL DISORDER

Claire is a former futures trader in her midforties who suffered from the disorder known as Persistent Genital Arousal Disorder (PGAD). This syndrome is completely unrelated to sex drive and probably involves compression and/or irritation of the pudendal nerve and inappropriate blood-vessel engorgement of the clitoral erectile tissue. The slightest touch sent Claire into arousal and sometimes orgasm, no matter where she was, or what she was doing.

"I would have given anything for this feeling to go away, and I would have rather never had an orgasm the rest of my life than to have this go on," she says. "I was totally ashamed and mortified, and would never tell anyone but my doctor and husband."

The condition affected her daily functioning in profound ways. "Every time I did something, I had to evaluate my situation: *Where am I? Are there other people around?* It was very disturbing to have this feeling of being aroused when you are around other people. It made me want to crawl under the covers and hide from people. Some people said how lucky I was to have those feelings. I felt like this was such a curse. I felt like I was suffering from some form of a perversion, even though I intellectually knew that it was medically rooted," Claire says.

"I would do anything to suppress an arousal, and when I felt one coming, I wanted to jump out of my skin. I would sometimes want to amputate my clitoris because I felt pain in that area would be preferable to the constant feeling of arousal."

Thankfully, PGAD is a condition that is generally quite treatable. With the help of the treatments discussed below, Claire has improved immensely, and is well on her way to enjoying her orgasms again.

COMMON MISDIAGNOSES
FOR CLITORAL PAIN AND PGAD

MISDIAGNOSIS	HOW TO RULE IT OUT
Recurrent genital herpes	Magnified exam of clitoris, herpes cultures, and blood test for herpes antibodies
Recurrent yeast infection	Wet smear, specific fungal culture, or DNA test
Recurrent urethra infection	Specific bacterial cultures
Genital warts	Magnified exam of clitoris
Psychological illness	MD awareness/education

DIAGNOSIS: THE TESTS YOU NEED

Chronic sexual pain is one of the most commonly misdiagnosed and mis-treated conditions in all of medicine. We've seen dozens of patients whose doctors didn't perform the correct diagnostic tests to properly identify their disorders—or, in some cases, didn't perform any tests at all but instead relied on a quick look. This section is to help you ensure that your physician is ordering the right tests to create a good diagnosis and treatment plan. If he or she is not ordering these tests, you probably want to consider finding another doctor.

First and foremost, your doctor needs to give you a good physical exam, delineating the area of tenderness, ruling out small abnormalities in the clitoris, and evaluating for muscle and nerve problems along the paths that might be the source of pain. The exam needs to include a detailed skin exam, with your physician looking closely at all the folds in your genitals with magnification, pulling back the clitoral hood for good exposure of all the surfaces. He or she will be looking for white areas, inflammation, ulceration, and injury, and should also be taking cultures to see if the area has been infected.

Your physician should also evaluate other parts of your pelvis and lower back to look for muscle spasms, hip disorders, and scarring of fascia and other connective tissue. You should be given a vaginal exam to rule out irritating vaginitis (since abnormal discharge might also affect your clitoris), and your doctor should take cultures for yeast, bacteria, and viruses.

Depending on your history and on the results of your physical exam, your doctor might want to do further imaging (such as MRIs) to test for abnormalities in blood-vessel, pelvic floor, and other pelvic structures. We believe strongly that pelvic floor muscle therapy is a crucial part of treatment for this type of pain, as well as for diagnosing possible orthopedic or muscular causes of the problem, so your doctor should almost always call for a physiatry or physical-therapy consultation to explore whether muscle imbalance and movement disorders might be affecting your clitoral nerves. He or she may also want to schedule a neurology consultation to evaluate for nerve compression and small-fiber neuropathy. (See Chapter 9 for more on testing for nerve problems.)

TREATMENTS: WHAT YOU CAN EXPECT

Here's the good news, and it is very good news indeed: Most cases of clitorodynia or persistent genital arousal can be cured. So please, please, please do not give up hope. Yes, the pain is excruciating, and the condition often seems as though it's taken over your life. But you can be helped, and the pain will go away. Rally your support system, and keep the ultimate goal in mind. This is an eminently treatable condition, and once you find a physician who knows how to treat you, help is on the way.

Effective treatment begins with identifying and then treating the underlying cause—which, as we have seen, might be anything from a skin condition to a muscular problem to a vascular issue to a nerve disorder, or some combination of many causes. Once the underlying cause or causes have been addressed, your physician should then move on to deal with the nerve sensitization that has almost certainly resulted from the pain itself.

Which treatments are appropriate will depend on the fundamental diagnosis, but the following are the most likely possibilities.

If your skin has been infected, you'll be given oral or topical antifungals or antibacterials to use for at least one month.

Your nerves may be desensitized with such topical nerve-sedating medications as lidocaine, bupivacaine, gabapentin (Neurontin), or amitriptyline (Elavil), to be applied frequently over the course of each day for three months.

If the regional nerves are the problem, you may be given a series of local anti-inflammatory and anesthetizing injections alongside the clitoris—at the clitoral branches of the pudendal nerve, at the pudendal nerve itself, or at one or more of the three neighboring nerve pathways.

In order to address the muscle and fascia tension and the tightness along these nerves in the pelvic floor and pelvis, physical therapy is a mainstay of any treatment. The nerves may become further irritated by the pelvic tightening and gripping that is a response to the pain—a vicious cycle.

If a blood-vessel abnormality is suspected, imaging and interventions to close off the culprit vessel are available.

If your problem is central nervous system pain or neuropathic (peripheral nerve injury) pain, you might be given oral medications (see Chapter 9).

If injured nerves are the problem, you might—in rare cases—be treated with pulsed radiofrequency (a method to "stun" the nerves) or sacral neuromodulation (see Chapter 9).

In severe cases, where the nerves do not respond to other treatments, nerve release surgery may be needed (see Chapter 9).

Persistent Genital Arousal Disorder is helped by all the treatments in this list and may also respond to medication and herbs that lower dopamine levels in the brain, such as varenicline (Chantix), risperidone, St. John's wort, and kava kava.

If an orthopedic injury is at the root of your problem, physical therapy that is focused on that injury can be very helpful. In extreme cases, you might need orthopedic surgical repair.

HOW *NOT* TO TREAT CLITORAL PAIN

Do *not* . . .

- pretend it does not really exist.

- listen to the opinions of people who aren't well informed or well educated about the condition.

- allow yourself to believe it's just in your head.

- use topical steroids without your physician's approval.

- decide that nothing could be worse than this and give up hope.

- avoid counseling to cope with this tough condition.

POTENTIAL BREAKTHROUGHS: LOOKING TOWARD THE FUTURE

We're happy to report that a great deal of very promising research is going on in nerve-pain and pain-biology science. As we understand more about nerves and about pain itself, we should be able to treat clitoral pain far more quickly and efficiently than we are now able to do. As new approaches are further developed, they'll become more available, and physicians will become more used to treating clitoral pain and PGAD. The medical silence surrounding this condition will be broken once and for all.

Meanwhile, if you're seeking or receiving treatment for this condition, be assured that things will get better. "After I started taking medication, I haven't had one moment with the thought that I can't live with this," Jessie says. Although she is still trying to determine whether she must resign herself to a certain degree of pain, she is far from hopeless. She says, "I now know I can do things to help myself."

8

PAIN AT THE
VAGINAL
OPENING

I never had any sexual problems. But I had been dating the same guy for quite a while, and one time, when we had intercourse, I suddenly had excruciating pain. We tried a couple more times to have sex after that first painful episode, and the pain stayed the same. That was when I knew I had a real problem.

—MIRIAM, HISTORY PROFESSOR, AGE THIRTY-THREE

I started feeling pain when I was a junior in college, when I put tampons in. Before this time, putting tampons in was never painful. So I went to my college health center, and they told me it was a yeast infection and gave me Diflucan. The Diflucan didn't do anything to help, so I went back, and they gave me creams, which also did nothing. . . . I couldn't understand what was wrong with me and why nobody could help.

—KELSEY, MARKETING EXECUTIVE FOR A DESIGNER
CLOTHING COMPANY, AGE TWENTY-SEVEN

I was raised in a traditional and religious home, so I didn't want to have sex until I met someone I truly loved. I had my first sexual encounter at age thirty-five. I had heard sex was supposed to be painful the first time. But the pain I felt was way over the top. I didn't think there was anything wrong with me psychologically, I just thought that because I waited so long, I was very tight. But I didn't get better.

—MELANIE, LIBRARIAN, AGE FORTY

I felt like I should be dating at this time in my life. But I felt like no man that I would meet would have ever heard of my problems. I kept thinking that a man would look down at that part of my body and be horrified that it is so red and inflamed. I hadn't had sex in so long, and I was petrified about what it would feel like. When I have had sex, I had terrible searing pain in my vaginal opening. I also have fissures and had to worry about sexual positions. I felt like I was damaged goods, and that no man would want to date me.

—THERESA, SPEECH THERAPIST, LATE TWENTIES

VESTIBULODYNIA: AN OVERVIEW

You might have felt it the first time you ever tried to have sex—and every time thereafter. Or you might have had a satisfying sex life for months or even years—and then suddenly felt burning pain every time someone or something entered you. Either way, you wonder why you're not able to enjoy penetration or even to tolerate it, and you're not sure which is worse, the excruciating pain or the tormenting doubts.

The medical term is vestibulodynia (pronounced ves-ti-byew-low-DIH-nia)—literally, pain at the vestibule, the opening of the vagina. We divide this condition into two categories: primary vestibulodynia, which we believe a woman is born with, and secondary vestibulodynia, which we assume a woman has acquired. But we think it might be a single condition with many variations and many possible causes: genetics, hormonal issues (including early use of the birth-control pill), nerve overgrowth, inflammation, and possible microtraumas to the vaginal opening. In any case, whether you've had this condition all your life or just developed it recently, the symptoms—and the treatment—are similar.

Primary vestibulodynia occurs during a woman's first experience of sexual activity that involves direct contact with the vaginal opening or even with the first attempt at insertion of a tampon. Pain might be caused by intercourse but also by manual stimulation, oral sex, and the use of dildos, vibrators, and sex toys. Secondary vestibulodynia can occur without warning at any point during a woman's sexual life, and when it appears, it involves the same type of pain. Together, the two conditions affect some 17 percent of all women at some time in their lives. Estimates put the number of U.S. women suffering now or in the past from this condition at almost twenty million.

WHAT'S GOING ON: THE BIOLOGY

The vestibule is a sexually sensitive part of the body, where touching, stroking, and contact with sex toys or with a penis can normally bring a lot of pleasure. It's also a generally sensitive area, because of the way that our different body parts come together there. Within the inner vaginal lips of the vulva, the vestibule is an "in between" place or a "border zone," where the membrane lining the inner walls of the vagina connects to the skin of the external female genitals.

Research shows that the vestibule exists here due to a capricious act of embryologic development. In the male fetus at two to three months, this same tissue becomes part of the penis's long inner urethral canal, through which urine is expelled from the body. In the female fetus, this tissue ends up as the vestibule but keeps all those "urethral"-type cells and behavior. So it is very responsive to hormones, as you'll read later in this chapter. Perhaps it is easily irritated because it works better as an inner lining to a tube, not as a surface that is out in the open.

To make matters more complex, within the vestibule are the hymen, the urethral opening, the periurethral (Skene's) and minor vestibular glands (involved in secretion of fluids with sexual arousal), and the ducts of the Bartholin's glands, which secrete mucus to add to vaginal lubrication (see illustrations 6-1 and 7-1). And these structures may become irritated and inflamed, magnifying the discomfort and pain, particularly during urination.

Pain in the vestibule used to be called vulvar vestibulitis, but the suffix "itis" in medicine usually connotes inflammation caused by infection (like tonsillitis), which does not seem to be a cause of this condition. The suffix "odynia" simply means "pain," so "vestibulodynia" is more appropriate. You might still hear the old-fashioned term, however, since—as with other causes of sexual pain—most medical professionals tend to be woefully out of touch with the latest research.

Scientists believe that primary vestibulodynia is probably present from birth. Certainly, many girls and young women have had lifelong difficulties in that area. Often, the vestibule is so sensitive that even putting in a tampon causes pain. Biopsies of girls and women with primary vestibulodynia usually show nerve overgrowth, also known as "sprouting" or "neuroprolifera-tion." The extra nerves become inflamed and oversensitive, causing pain.

Scientists likewise believe that secondary vestibulodynia appears later in life because of some kind of harm or injury to the vaginal area. The body responds, apparently, by generating the same kind of nerve overgrowth and inflammation experienced by women who have primary vestibulodynia.

Despite their different origins, the two conditions seem virtually identi-cal—which has led researchers to speculate that perhaps instead of multiple disorders, there is one continuum. The latest research suggests that women might be born with a genetic predisposition for this condition, which is then set off by some kind of trauma in the vaginal area, provoking the nerve overgrowth and the inflammation. Alternately, inflammation may create problems in the vestibule, which in turn provokes nerve overgrowth. Possibly, both explanations are correct: In some women, nerve overgrowth and the chemicals these nerves release provoke inflammation; in other women, inflammation provokes nerve overgrowth. Now, we only know that some women seem to have the condition from the first time they try to insert a tampon, and other women have a pain-free sex life for years and then develop the condition.

Unlike most other types of sexual pain, vestibulodynia leaves most women free from discomfort unless the vestibule is provoked by touch. Sometimes, though, if you keep trying to have sex, the area becomes further irritated and inflamed. In that case, you might also feel pain at other times, such as when you ride a bike, wear tight pants, sit for a long time, or do anything to put further pressure on the area.

If you first experienced pain when trying to use a tampon, you might have noticed that you felt fine once the tampon was in, but that it hurt again when you tried to take it out. That's because your vestibule—your vaginal opening—has that overgrowth of extra nerves, which become inflamed and irritated. So any passage over the vestibule brings discomfort or pain.

If you developed vestibulodynia as a teenager, you may not have understood why your first few sexual experiences were so painful. You might have believed—or been told—that if you just kept trying, you would get used to it—that you would "learn to relax" and start enjoying sex. You might even have been convinced that you had some kind of psychological problem rather than an identifiable physical condition.

If you developed this condition after enjoying pain-free sex, you might also have wondered whether it was a psychological problem. Many of our patients have told us that they started questioning themselves, their partners, and their relationships, since the pain began so suddenly and mysteriously, and since their physicians were not aware that this is a medical condition.

Unfortunately, if you have vestibulodynia, the more often you try to have sex, the more your body reflexively tenses to resist the pain. Often, the pelvic floor muscles and fascia become firm and tight around the vaginal opening, making sex even more difficult and, as you keep trying, more painful. Many unconsummated marriages are the result of this type of sexual problem.

Dispelling the Myth of "Frigidity"

This condition has probably been around for centuries, leading women to be labeled "frigid," or more recently, to be given the outdated diagnosis of "vaginismus." Named in the midnineteenth century, vaginismus was supposed to indicate spasms and clenching of the vagina, so that a penis could not enter. Founder of psychoanalysis Sigmund Freud believed the disorder signified women's anxieties about sex and their unwillingness to accept their female nature. Remarkably, this pseudoscientific diagnosis is still being given, and you can still find it even on otherwise reputable medical sites on the Internet. We personally believe that what has mistakenly been labeled vaginismus is most often some form of vestibulodynia, made worse by the muscle dysfunction coming either independently or as a stress response to sexual pain. (For more on muscle dysfunction and sexual pain, see Chapter 10.)

Pain during penetration is profoundly upsetting, whether you have developed it only recently or have never known anything else. We want to assure you in no uncertain terms that you are suffering from a medical condition—overgrowth of nerves in a sensitive area—and that the right medical treatment can free you from this pain. Almost certainly, if sex is or has become painful, you are now struggling with psychological issues as well, as you try to come to terms with why you can't enjoy a part of life that others seem to find so pleasurable. But those issues are not the cause of your medical condition—they are the result. When you clear up the medical problem—which is entirely within the reach of current medical science—you'll be able to experience comfortable sex.

Possible Causes and Factors

We're still trying to grasp the reasons behind this painful condition, and there's a lot we don't yet know. Vestibular skin is different from both regular skin and vaginal mucous membranes; it bears a strong resemblance to urethral canal tissue. As a result of the special nature of vestibular skin, it may be thinner and less elastic than other body surfaces, which makes it more susceptible to trauma or microscopic tears and which makes it take longer to heal. Vestibular skin seems to have extra nerve endings, which perhaps can become more easily overgrown. It also seems to include numerous cell receptors for estrogen, testosterone, and progesterone, which makes it unusually responsive to hormonal changes and other systemwide conditions in the body.

HORMONES

We've had patients who immediately felt better after going off the birth-control pill, and some research suggests that early use of the pill might be responsible for the condition in some young women, or that it might trigger their genetic predispositions to it. The Pill reduces levels of ovarian estrogen and testosterone, which participate in the normal functioning of vestibular cells, so perhaps vestibulodynia and inflamed nerves are somehow a response to "hungry" receptors on vestibular cells, seeking the hormones they are deprived of. When our tissues lack the stimulatory hormonal "fuel" they need, they thin or "atrophy," and because vestibular tissue is especially rich in hormone receptors, it may be especially "needy." (If you have pain upon intercourse and penetration, and you're undergoing menopause or another major hormonal change, you should read Chapter 13, since your problem probably has less to do with overgrown nerve endings and inflammation and more to do with hormonal issues.)

GENETICS

We suspect that vestibulodynia has genetic roots. We've seen identical twins with the same condition, so possibly, some women are born either with the condition or with a vulnerability to it. Or, like other pain syndromes, the disorder may be a developmental response to medical or emotional trauma that affected pain processing in the womb, in infancy (such as neonatal intensive-care stay) or early childhood (for women diagnosed with primary vestibulodynia), or even later (for women diagnosed with secondary vestibulodynia). There is growing evidence that intense physical pain experiences, especially early in life, alter processing of future sensations, but remember these are physical responses in the nervous system itself, not emotional reactions.

EARLY INJURY

Some European researchers believe that vestibulodynia results from a lack of arousal when a woman has intercourse for the first time, leading to pain from insufficient lubrication and from reflexive gripping of the muscles at the vaginal opening. A woman would be especially likely to be dry and tense if she were feeling anxious, or if her first sexual experience didn't include enough stimulation, comfort, and gentleness. As a result, penetration might cause small tears in the vestibule, the hymen, and the hymenal remnants (small mucosal tags that remain at the vaginal opening for life once the hymen itself has been opened with penetration). This tissue in the majority of women would heal well, but in those who may be genetically predisposed to inflammation, the tissue injury might lead to local inflammation, nerve sensitization, and ongoing pain every time something crosses her vestibule.

NERVE IRRITATION AND INFLAMMATION: A VICIOUS CIRCLE

Another theory is that women with primary vestibulodynia are born with more nerve endings than normal, with many dense, sprouted "nerve branches" growing in a fine weave. These nerve endings bring in more inflammatory cells, such as mast cells, which are normally part of the body's immune response but which can trigger negative side effects, such as redness, swelling, heat, and pain. Mast cells also release cytokines and histamines, immune-system chemicals that can also irritate and inflame an area. They even make a substance called nerve growth factor (NGF), which stimulates the sprouting of even more nerve endings. The chemical cascade becomes a vicious circle, with the nerve irritation and inflammation feeding on itself.

Women with secondary vestibulodynia have probably suffered a tissue trauma or injury that brings inflammatory chemicals to the area. The chemical cascade then provokes an overgrowth of more nerves. Our patients have reported that their vestibulodynia appeared soon after the following triggers:

- the prolonged consumption of oral antibiotics;

- diarrhea, which can irritate and inflame the whole vulvar and vestibular area;

- taking the birth-control pill for more than two years;

- a chronic yeast infection (though this may have been a misdiagnosis);

- a new sexual relationship, perhaps with more sexual activity, or a partner with a larger penis;

- a different use of sex toys;

- using a douche or other over-the-counter treatment;

- a severe flare-up of genital herpes;

- severe mold infestation at home;

- a new job with prolonged sitting;

- exposure to or prolonged use of an over-the-counter topical cream;

- a bad allergy season or asthma exacerbation severe enough to require steroid medication and decongestants, which are drying agents;

- hormone imbalances or changes, including weight loss, associated with amenorrhea or menstrual irregularity, and menopause (see Chapter 13); or

- a flare-up of eczema or other inflammatory or allergic skin conditions elsewhere on the body.

ALLERGIC AND AUTOIMMUNE RESPONSES

Cases like those just mentioned have caused scientists to wonder whether autoimmune or allergic factors might also contribute to the condition. Allergies are a kind of autoimmune reaction, in which mast cells and other immune-system chemicals mobilize in response to a perceived threat— a chemical that you ingested, inhaled, or put on your skin. In fact, many women with vestibulodynia have a history of respiratory and skin allergies, suggesting that the inflammation response occurs in many places throughout the body.

You might also develop the condition—or make it worse—through an allergic or contact reaction to a cream or ointment applied to the area. Even after the initial irritant is taken away, the inflammation may continue and snowball.

INFECTIONS

Fungal infections, including yeast infections, may also be part of the problem, as the chemicals that these organisms release damage the vestibular tissue and nerve endings. Although most women with yeast infections never develop vestibular problems, repeated yeast infections might be an issue for some women, either creating the problem, triggering an allergy to yeast, or preventing an existing condition from quieting down.

To make matters still worse, the topical chemicals used to treat yeast infections might further inflame the area. So now you're in pain because of inflamed nerve endings, additional inflammatory chemicals, a yeast infection, *and* the chemicals used to treat the yeast infection. It can feel overwhelming, to say the least.

SYMPTOMS OF VESTIBULODYNIA

If you are suffering from vestibulodynia, you are likely to have one or more of the following symptoms:

- burning, stinging, itching, or throbbing as a result of touch at your vaginal opening;

- numbness as a result of continued touching or penetration;

- after touching or penetration, a residual afterburn or itching that can last from minutes to days;

- with repeated attempts at penetration, a swelling, tearing, or cutting sensation around the vaginal opening, especially in the V-shaped section at the back (called the posterior fourchette); and/or

- persistent urethral burning after sex or during or after urinating—this may be the main symptom of vestibulodynia in some women (the urethra's opening is part of the vestibule and is made of the same tissue).

HOW VESTIBULODYNIA AFFECTS YOU

Many women are profoundly confused by pain at the vaginal opening, especially if they develop it later in life, after a time of being able to enjoy touching and penetration in this area. If you try to look at the area yourself, it will probably appear normal, or perhaps mildly red, though you may see rawness or cracking at the back of the vestibule. You may believe you've got some kind of skin irritation, or perhaps a yeast infection. Many of our patients tried one over-the-counter remedy after another to address what they thought was the problem, but most creams and ointments will only make the problem worse.

Meanwhile, whether you've had this condition all your life or only recently developed it, you are almost certainly plagued by anxiety and despair. You wonder why you can't have a normal sex life, or what is so wrong with you that you are "resisting" sex. You may begin to believe that you're psychologically damaged, "frigid," or unwilling to accept your identity as a woman. You are very likely to get advice and diagnoses—even from doctors and therapists—that are simply incorrect and that make you feel even worse.

COMMON MISDIAGNOSES FOR VESTIBULODYNIA

MISDIAGNOSIS	HOW TO RULE IT OUT
Recurrent genital herpes	Magnified exam of the vestibule, herpes cultures, blood test for herpes antibodies
Recurrent yeast infection	Wet smear, specific fungal culture, or DNA test
Recurrent bladder/ urethra infection	Specific bacterial cultures
Genital warts	Magnified exam of vestibule
Painful bladder syndrome	Often coexist; cystoscopy
Vaginismus	Magnified exam and pelvic floor exam
Psychological illness	MD awareness/education

SHADES OF PAIN

Sex and pain are highly subjective topics for most women, and each of our patients with vestibulodynia describes her symptoms in her own way:

- "horrible burning at the opening of my vagina"

- "a hot and raw feeling that itches sometimes"

- "sharp pain, like a knife or a hot poker stabbing my vagina"

- "a numbness in my vagina that develops during my husband's thrusts when we have intercourse"

- "vaginal pain that lasts for hours, or sometimes even days, after I've had sex"

If you are in a relationship, you may feel anxious, guilty, angry, or depressed about not being able to have certain kinds of sex with your partner. If you are single, you may worry that you'll never be able to find anyone who will tolerate your problem—or you may worry that you won't even be able to explain to anyone what's wrong with you. Whether you're single or partnered, you may worry about your sexual and romantic future, and may fear your condition will never improve.

If you are diagnosed with primary vestibulodynia before you've been sexually active, you may feel betrayed, anxious, and confused about what sex will be like for you. "Until the point I was diagnosed, I never had a serious relationship, and I had never been sexually active," Kelsey says. "If I had been sexually active at sixteen or seventeen, I would not have been as upset. I wanted a boyfriend really badly in college, but I just didn't have one. I really felt jilted by my whole college experience. I never had college hookups, and I am sad about that."

You may also feel so upset about your condition that you simply shut down. "When I was really bummed out, I stayed home and hid," admits Theresa. "And if my friends were doing something physical, like going out for a run, I gracefully bowed out. Sometimes I was so anxious I couldn't sleep, and sometimes I woke up in a panic. Sometimes I coped with the whole thing by eating—overeating, really. I had always been a very physical person and very health-conscious. But it seemed like food was the only thing I could count on not to hurt."

Note: Some 70 percent of the time, vestibulodynia coexists with urethral syndrome (burning pain in the lower portion of the urethra), painful bladder syndrome, irritable bowel syndrome, or pelvic floor muscle dysfunction.

DIAGNOSIS: THE TESTS YOU NEED

Chronic sexual pain is one of the most commonly misdiagnosed and mistreated conditions in all of medicine. We've seen dozens of patients whose doctors didn't perform the correct diagnostic tests to properly identify their disorders—or, in some cases, didn't perform any tests at all but instead relied on a quick look. This section is to help you ensure that your physician is ordering the right tests to create a good diagnosis and treatment plan. If he or she is not ordering these tests, you probably want to consider finding another doctor.

The first thing you need is a good physical exam, conducted with magnification. Some of the following signs should be visible, but they can be subtle, so your doctor should look for them carefully:

- pink to red to purplish overall color of the vestibule;

- mottled color of the vestibule, due to the visibility of small blood vessels under the thinned surface;

- areas of deeper red at the openings of the Bartholin's glands and minor vestibular glands in the crevices next to the hymen (see illustrations 6-1 and 7-1);

- overall thinning of the vestibule;

- tiny fissures, cracks, or erosions in the V at the back of the vestibule, known as the posterior fourchette; or

- redness, abrasions, and swelling of the hymen.

The "Q-tip test" is also useful to identify where and how pain occurs. Your physician should touch a Q-tip with uniform pressure gently to differ- ent parts of your vestibule and hymen, and then, for comparison, to other areas of the vulva. The gentle touch should elicit the burning, sharpness, and pinlike sensations that are evidence of vestibulodynia.

Likewise, an exam with fingers touching the area should also elicit ten- derness. A digital (finger) exam will often also reveal inelastic surface tissue, as well as restricted underlying fascia and other connective tissue at the base of the vestibule.

Your doctor should also determine whether there are any related problems that might be causing you additional sexual pain, especially with regard to your pelvic floor muscles and fascia (see Chapter 10). In fact, this is another reason why treatment of vestibulodynia is so crucial, because, left untreated, it tends to progress: First, there's pain in the vestibule upon touching or penetration. Then, when the woman tenses her muscles against the pain, she might develop spasms, pain, and shortening in her pelvic floor muscles. The muscle response creates pressure on the bladder and additional pain (see Chapter 12), and also can compress the pudendal nerve, causing yet more pain (see Chapter 9). But when caught and treated early, the pain and symptoms may be completely confined to the vestibule, so we can put our therapeutic focus there.

DON'T LET YOUR PHYSICIAN CAUSE YOU PAIN!

If your exam is painful at any point, tell your doctor—when and how you feel pain is an important diagnostic clue. If your exam becomes too painful, ask the doctor to stop that portion of it. There is no reason for you to suffer while being examined, and trying to "tough it out" may actually delay or reverse your healing.

Our patient Miriam had a ghastly encounter with a gynecologist who had years of experience treating women—but not with sexual pain:

> I thought I was going to die during the exam. I don't know what she did, but she definitely used instruments that weren't right for people with my condition. I remember lying on the exam table, and I was in such terrible pain, and I have a very high pain tolerance. I began to think that this woman was out of her mind. She didn't even examine the spot where I had pain. I said to the doctor, "With all due respect, if you don't take that speculum out of me I think I am going to hit you."
>
> The doctor then said to me, "You are a little tense."
>
> I said to her, "Are you out of your mind? I came to you because I am in such pain, and you put me through this excruciating pain, and you are telling me I am a little tense?!"
>
> Instead of trying to find out what was wrong with me from other sources or colleagues, she told me to have a sip of wine. This doctor didn't even have a clue if I was an alcoholic, and she is telling me to drink alcohol!

Don't endure what Miriam did. If your doctor cannot examine you with sensitivity and respect, find another doctor.

TREATMENTS: WHAT YOU CAN EXPECT

As it is so often with sexual pain, we have both good news and bad news about the treatments. The bad news is that it may take a while to work through all the related issues and to discover the treatment that will ultimately be effective. The good news, though, is that there are many approaches we can try, and there's lots of room to be optimistic about a full, complete recovery from this painful condition.

Our usual plan is to start with the simplest and safest treatments, especially because they often get good results, and the problem can stop right there. If not, there are more complex and demanding treatments that we can try, so we work our way down the list of possibilities. There are also some things you can do right away to protect and strengthen your vestibule.

Protecting Your Vestibule

Usually it takes three to six months of treatment before you find yourself feeling better. However, there are some things you can do right away that will bring some immediate relief.

- Follow the genital wellness suggestions in Chapter 4.

- Delay attempts at intercourse or penetration for as long as you need to.

- Since fungi (yeast) such as *Candida* are major toxins to the vestibule, you might try weekly preventative antifungal therapy with oral fluconazole.

- Take a daily oral probiotic supplement, and ask your doctor about vaginal probiotics as well.

- Try acupuncture, which can help you tone down your reactions to touch in the genital area and which can help relax your central nervous system (see Chapter 4).

Strengthening Your Vestibule

As we have seen, your vestibular tissue tends to become very thin in this condition, allowing for more irritation of the plethora of overgrown nerves just under the surface. Since hormonal issues may be involved, stopping the birth-control pill may be extremely helpful. You might be able to start again once your healing is complete.

We do not give this advice lightly, because the Pill in other ways has been so liberating for women's sexuality since it was introduced in the 1960s. Also, the Pill has been proven to decrease the risk of ovarian cancer, uterine cancer, endometriosis, ovarian cysts, osteoporosis, and painful and heavy menstrual periods. The good news is that we do now have several other effective treatments for heavy, painful, and irregular menses, if that is why you are taking the Pill. As one example, a new medication called tranexamic acid (Lysteda) works well to reduce heavy flow. But if stopping the Pill is too worrisome to you, you may be able to keep taking it if your doctor is able to compensate by prescribing topical hormonal creams to apply to your vestibule.

Contact with irritants might also be a risk, so follow the advice in Chapter 4, which might strengthen your vestibule even if you're still on the Pill.

Compounded low-dose hormonal creams and oils available in various hypoallergenic bases can help strengthen the surface of the vestibule. The best combination usually includes bioidentical estradiol or estriol and testosterone. Specially trained compounding pharmacists have the expertise to place these hormones in a variety of bases that are nonirritating and hypoallergenic, much better for your already delicate vestibule than the pharmaceutically manufactured creams such as Estrace and Premarin cream, which have additives. You'll likely see a benefit within one to two months. (See the Resources section at the back of the book for recommended high-quality compounding pharmacies.)

Treating the "Sprouted" Abnormal Nerve Endings

You can begin taking supplements right away to help restore and maintain the health of your nerves. See "Nourish your nerves and your body" in Chapter 4 for some suggestions. Ice packs are a good temporary nerve sedative for pain flares. In Deborah's office, the staff freeze water-filled condoms to use as ice packs for the vestibule.

Once the surface of your vestibule is stronger, topical medications may help calm the nerves. You might be prescribed liquid lidocaine or bupivacaine without additives; a cotton ball is soaked in the medication and placed as a patch on the vestibule overnight. You might be prescribed amitriptyline (Elavil) or gabapentin (Neurontin) ointment, or similar medication, to be taken for two to three months (in some advanced cases, your doctor may also prescribe oral versions of these medications).

Using Physical Therapy to Open Up the Area

We can't stress it enough: Physical therapy is essential for treating pain in the vestibule. You want to mobilize the soft tissues in the area, to elongate the restricted fascia and other connective tissue under the surface and around the nerve endings, and to improve blood supply to the nerves for healing. Please work with a physical therapist, and do the exercises you are given. We have seen patients avoid physical therapy for various reasons, and they progress so slowly compared to those who fully take on this treatment.

One key aspect of physical therapy for your condition is the use of dilators—long tubes of varying thicknesses that are inserted into your vagina, training your vestibule to experience penetration and encouraging your vaginal muscles to relax, rest, and elongate. Typically, a very small tube is used at first, moving on to thicker and thicker tubes that match the size of a penis or sex toy. Working with dilators will help your pelvic muscles grow longer and help you to relax them after so many months or years of clenching them against the pain. This type of physical therapy can also help build your confidence in your ability to be penetrated (see "Vaginal Dilator" section in

Chapter 10). And the more you know about what's going on in your own anatomy, the more empowered and confident you will feel.

Treating Chronic Inflammation

Because histamines and other inflammatory chemicals are involved in this condition, your doctor may prescribe oral medications such as hydroxyzine (an antihistamine that suppresses the function of the mast cells), or montelukast (Singulair) or topical cromolyn sodium, both of which inhibit other irritating chemicals. Some of these medications can make you drowsy, so you're likely to take them at bedtime.

Treating the Muscles around the Vestibule

If after three to six months you've gotten no significant relief from treating the vestibule itself, your doctor may move to treat the muscles around the area, whose tension may be perpetuating your pain. He or she may use dry-needling: inserting a very thin needle into the muscle—almost as thin as an acupuncture needle—and moving the needle in and out. No medication is involved, just the needle itself. Remarkably, your muscle relaxes immediately—and this relaxation brings a great deal of relief. Trigger-point injections are similar—a trigger point, which is a portion of a pelvic floor muscle that when touched causes tightening and contraction of a wider area of muscle, is injected with a small amount of anesthetic medication. This can decrease the overall tension of the pelvic floor.

Some patients find that these injections bring only temporary relief. In that case, your doctor may administer injections of botulinum toxin A (Botox) to specific contracted and tender muscles under your vestibule, which may allow them to remain released for up to three months.

Your doctor should also re-examine you for other types of pelvic floor muscle problems and pudendal nerve irritation, and should treat you for those disorders as needed.

Surgical Treatments

Most women don't need surgical treatment, but various types are available for the few who do. The least invasive type is minor surgical revisions for what physicians call "localized stubbornly painful areas," such as the small chronic fissures—like paper cuts—that occur in the posterior fourchette. That's because, with each penetration, the scarred thin tissue retears, then heals over the next three to four days, then retears again with intercourse. Usually, physical therapy helps bring flexibility to the inelastic fascia while improving blood supply. In some cases, though, removal of the small scarred areas is very helpful. This is actually an office procedure—no hospitalization needed.

Another office procedure is the removal of tender, swollen, tearing hymenal remnants that pull on the vestibular tissue with penetration, and that burn with contact. This procedure can often take a major portion of inflammation away and can help the vestibule respond to other treatments.

The next level of surgery is vestibulectomy, removal of the vestibule itself. It is also available as the more minor "modified posterior vestibulectomy" for those women who have pain only at the bottom of the vestibule, around the posterior fourchette. In our experience, though, most women who require surgery need the larger procedure, known as a "total vestibulectomy with vaginal advancement."

The total vestibulectomy involves removing most of the abnormal surface, along with the underlying nerve endings and inflammatory tissue. It is best performed under general anesthesia. Because you need at least three months to heal from this surgery, and you won't be able to sit down comfortably for extended periods of time for six weeks afterward, we look to this surgery as a kind of last resort after treating any coexisting problems with skin, nerves, and muscles. Fortunately, most women don't need the procedure.

If you do have the surgery, your three-month healing period will be difficult. Even a menstrual pad will be painful, and you certainly won't feel like having sex. You will definitely need to undertake physical therapy and use dilators. We strongly recommend getting your pelvic area into good physical shape before surgery, so that everything is strong and "ready to go" afterward.

Surgery seems to be most effective in women with primary vestibulo-dynia. In most studies, improvement rates are close to 85 percent if patients are properly selected. However, as of this writing, we doctors in the field don't yet have complete, organized data for outcome analysis. Studies from Israel—where a great deal of sexual-pain research has been done for years—suggest that vestibulectomy is a good treatment, but that only about 60 per-cent of all women have a complete cure, though some 85 percent get better at least partially.

Cosmetically, at least, the results are excellent. Only a doctor would notice an anatomical difference. Rarely, women may have small areas of residual vestibule tissue remaining behind and therefore pain persistence at that site after the surgery (often at the urethral opening). This can often be corrected with small excisions of the painful spots done as an office procedure.

HOW *NOT* TO TREAT VESTIBULAR PAIN

Do *not* . . .

- ignore diarrhea that may be irritating the vestibular skin.

- apply any substance if you haven't read the list of ingredients.

- apply anything that contains propylene glycol, ben-zocaine, parabens, or other chemicals. If you have not heard of a listed additive, cannot pronounce it,

➤

> or cannot read it because it is in a foreign language, chances are high that it is not good for your genital skin! And products made in China often have unlisted toxic ingredients. The simpler the product the better.

- apply topical steroids on your own without your physician's advice.

- take bubble baths (oatmeal baths are the only ones that may help).

- apply antifungal topical treatments unless your physician has specifically tested for and found a yeast infection (if you don't have one, antifungals can make things worse).

- take any type of antibiotic, whether oral or topical, without consulting a physician (it could worsen your condition, cause painful side effects, and make you resistant to antibiotics, making treatment of future infections more difficult).

- resort to older forms of laser treatments—research has shown them to be inadequate.

- jump to surgery without trying less-severe treatments.

- ignore coexisting conditions that need treatment also for full recovery.

- force yourself to have intercourse if you're not yet ready during your treatment.

POTENTIAL BREAKTHROUGHS: LOOKING TOWARD THE FUTURE

The very good news about vestibulodynia is that it is very treatable. Once you've gotten it under control, it usually stays under control, and even if you do have a flare-up, you can almost always go back to what has helped in the past and see immediate results. Sometimes hormonal changes will produce another flare-up, and then you may need to resume the application of hormone creams, get off the Pill, or do whatever worked before. During menopause, you may also want to consider additional treatment (see Chapter 13). But for the most part, you can expect you will be able to treat this condition and resume—or begin—a normal sex life.

Meanwhile, new diagnostic tests, nerve research, and research into inflammation are helping us to understand this confusing condition, so there is a lot of room for optimism. Current studies are focusing on such topics as how to pick the right candidates for surgery; how to strengthen the tissues with a new use of lasers, other energy sources, and injectables; and how to prevent this all-too-common sexual pain from happening in the first place.

Our patients with vestibulodynia have gone on to satisfying lives. Kelsey, who finally had a vestibulectomy, was relieved to be able to have sex after that, though she still needs to be cautious sometimes. Of her life with her new boyfriend, she says, "I think we have found a way to keep our intimacy. He knows what's uncomfortable for me, and if I say something is uncomfortable, he backs off, so I never feel pressured. He also loves cuddling, and he said he never did that before me. I think we really have a good bond."

Melanie and her partner have also learned to work around her condition. "I still have some pain during sex, but it is better," she says. "I have to wait a few days between having sex. In the beginning of each time we have sex, the penetration hurts, so what I do is try to find a position that accommodates me so I don't feel as much pain. We do a lot of foreplay—that's the key. And when we feel he is ready, we make sure penetration is at the point where he doesn't have to stay in too long."

Both Miriam and Theresa have been happy with their recoveries. When we ask Theresa how she's doing, she simply smiles and says, "Pain is no longer a big part of my life. And I found a great guy who loves me for who I am!"

9

.....

NERVE PAIN

I first noticed some burning during sexual intercourse. I continued to have sex even though I had pain, because I was in a state of denial. I thought I probably had an infection and that the pain would stop. But it just got worse and worse.

At this point, my husband and I can never have sexual intercourse. We try to be sexual by doing things other than intercourse. But even then, I still have pain with touching. Too much pressure on my vulva causes me additional pain. It feels like the top layers of my skin are being ripped off.

—SANDRA, BIOMEDICAL TECHNICIAN, AGE THIRTY-THREE

I have pain 24/7. I have a burning, raw, and itching feeling on the right side of my vulva. I also feel pain in my rectum and around my anus. The pain in my vulva on the right side is so intense—the labia burns, and it is so raw and itches so badly that I can't stand, sit, or walk. The pain also radiates down my thighs. Sex has become secondary because I am always in pain.

—LYNN, RETIRED TEACHER, LATE FIFTIES

NERVE PAIN: AN OVERVIEW

You feel burning, irritation, or itchiness in the skin of your vulva—either on the left side, the right side, or both. The sensations are so intense and uncomfortable, you can barely stand it, but there's no skin condition to explain your pain. Nothing down there looks different. But you're in constant discomfort, maybe even in constant pain. Not being able to understand what's happening or why is almost worse than the pain itself.

You may have been to a number of doctors who told you that this condition is "all in your head," but it isn't. You're suffering from either nerve damage, nerve inflammation, or the compression of one or more key nerves. Many doctors are now of the opinion that chronic vulvar nerve–type pain, also known as vulvodynia, is really one of the complex regional pain syndromes (CRPS) better recognized in other areas of the body. CRPS consists of pain in one area of the body (regional) that involves many different aspects of the nervous system (complex). We hope this term will replace the word vulvodynia soon, because it clarifies what is really going on: a complicated interaction of nerves in a particular region of the body, rather than a mysterious, ill-defined problem of the vulva.

As we saw in Chapter 5, the nervous system is made up of three major components, the peripheral nervous system, the autonomic nervous system, and the central nervous system. A disorder in any one of these systems could initially create pelvic and sexual pain, with all three systems somehow becoming involved in keeping the pain going in ways we don't fully understand.

One of the mysteries of nerve pain is the way it can continue after its ostensible source is gone. For example, a wound or trauma creates pain—but the pain persists even after the wound is healed or the trauma is long in the past. It's as though the nerves "learn" to transmit pain signals and then can't "unlearn" to do so without a lot of help.

This phenomenon has been observed in many regions of the body, most notably in the limbs and most dramatically in phantom-limb pain, where pain persists in the space where an amputated limb used to be, even though the nerve itself has been cut and is now missing. Because of the intimate and intense nature of sexual pain, and because of the specific ways in which it is processed by the brain, it may be even more difficult to bear.

The biology of chronic pain is a relatively new area of research in medical science, and we're rapidly learning more. The good news is that even without a full understanding of how this all works, we can do a lot to address this condition—and to relieve your pain. Although a doctor may not be able to see or measure your distress, your pain began as a biological experience, not a psychological one, and it can be medically treated.

SYMPTOMS OF NERVE PAIN

The following are symptoms of nerve-related sexual pain:

- burning, irritation, or itchiness of the vulvar skin (on either or both sides), without the presence of a skin condition or any other visual indicators;

- pain in the area where the pudendal nerve is responsible for sensation (the vulva, or in the "sensory area" of one of the three main pudendal nerve branches, in the anus, labia, or clitoris);

- pain often made worse by touch (including contact with clothing seams or by wiping after defecating); sustained sitting or activities like bike-riding are often too painful to endure;

- flares of high-intensity pain caused by even a light touch and lasting from hours to days; or

- sudden sharp, lacerating pain in the vaginal area, becoming worse with sitting or touch, and mostly constant.

COMMON MISDIAGNOSES
FOR PUDENDAL AND OTHER NERVE PAIN

MISDIAGNOSIS	HOW TO RULE IT OUT
Recurrent yeast infection	Wet smear, specific fungal culture or DNA test
Vulvar skin disorders (i.e., LSC)	Magnified vulvar exam, skin biopsy
Recurrent genital herpes	Magnified vulvar exam, herpes cultures, and blood test for herpes antibodies
Painful bladder syndrome	Often coexist; cystoscopy
Endometriosis	Pelvic exam, imaging studies, laparoscopy
Ovarian cysts	Pelvic exam, ultrasound
Psychological illness	MD awareness/education

HOW NERVE PAIN AFFECTS YOU

The most insidious aspect of nerve pain is the apparent lack of a reason for it. Many women feel anxiety or despair about intense, persistent pain whose source simply cannot be identified—especially if physicians, therapists, and loved ones believe that the problem is exaggerated or that its origins are "all in your head." Without medical confirmation or explanation of your experience, it can be all too easy to believe that your own attitudes or emotions are the source of your problem—a psychological self-punishment that can make the pain feel even worse.

Another danger of this type of pain is a problem for all types of pain: You tend to stop using the muscles associated with the painful area, and to retreat from activity generally. While this is an understandable reaction, it usually makes the problem worse. Not using your muscles means that they atrophy and become weak, which means that any muscular activity in the painful area is likely to cause even more pain. Likewise, if your understandable response to nerve pain is to clench or tighten your pelvic floor muscles, you are potentially creating pelvic floor dysfunction, giving yourself a second cause of sexual pain (see Chapter 10).

Of all the types of sexual pain, nerve pain is perhaps the most debilitating because of its intensity, its persistence, and its resistance to treatment. "There have been times when I just felt like I couldn't cope anymore, and I just wanted to die," Lynn says. "I felt like it just wasn't worth going on. I felt like there was no cure, no answers—and I just couldn't bear the thought of living like this anymore. Honestly, I don't know how I coped."

WHAT'S GOING ON: THE BIOLOGY

As we saw in Chapter 5, a normal nervous system transmits sensory impulses and does not overreact, itch for no reason, or generate its own pain. Yet if you're suffering from nerve pain, your nervous system is doing one or more of those things as the result of one or more of the following.

Pudendal Nerve Damage or Compression

Problems can occur anywhere along the long pudendal nerve, which extends from your lower spine through your pelvis and into your vulva [see illustration 9-1 for its three main branches, which may go by varied names: dorsal (clitoral), perineal (labial), and inferior hemorrhoidal (rectal)]. The pudendal nerve can become distressed in a wide variety of ways: irritation, inflammation, entrapment, or compression. Although a specific incident probably set the pain in motion, nerve pain often seems to continue of its own accord. In other types of pain, we treat or remove the cause—for example, we get a wound or a broken bone to heal. With nerve pain, we must address the nerves themselves, since the trauma that set them off is usually long over. Traumas that might set off continuing sexual

Illustration 9-1.

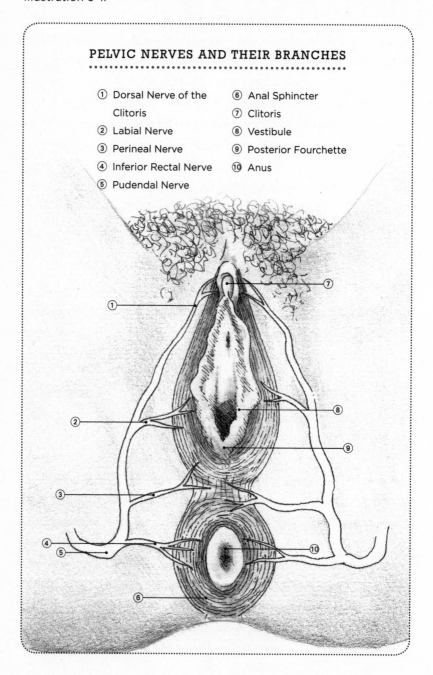

PELVIC NERVES AND THEIR BRANCHES

① Dorsal Nerve of the Clitoris
② Labial Nerve
③ Perineal Nerve
④ Inferior Rectal Nerve
⑤ Pudendal Nerve
⑥ Anal Sphincter
⑦ Clitoris
⑧ Vestibule
⑨ Posterior Fourchette
⑩ Anus

pain include bike-riding, childbirth, prolonged sitting, and changes in the muscles of the pelvic floor (see Chapter 10).

Pudendal neuralgia (also called neuritis and neuropathy) is any injury of the pudendal nerve that creates pain or dysfunction, either constant or intermittent. It is a common and very much underestimated source of sexual pain. It may be caused by compression of the pudendal nerve by muscle, fascia, other connective tissue, or scar tissue. The resulting damage may occur anywhere along the pudendal nerve's long journey from the lower spine (where at least three nerve roots from the sacrum combine to form that nerve) to the vulvar skin. Even if the nerve damage or compression occurs further up the nerve (for example, close to its exit from the spinal cord), the pain itself may be experienced as coming from the skin. In our experience, when a patient is given the diagnosis of "generalized vulvodynia" (generalized vulvar pain), a damaged, inflamed, or compressed pudendal nerve is usually involved.

Damage or Compression of Other Pelvic Nerves

Injury to any nerves that exit the spine and travel down in to the pelvic area can trigger sexual pain, including low-back injuries and surgery, as well as cesarean-delivery incisions.

The ilioinguinal and iliohypogastric nerves arise from the high lumbar spine at your waist and run around your body and down to your groin, pubic bone, and clitoris (see illustrations 5-1 and 7-1 for an idea of their anatomy). Irritation anywhere along their paths may cause pain in the top part of the vulva. Another vulnerable nerve is the genitofemoral, which runs along the psoas (a muscle that supports your spine and inserts into your groin). Inflammation, injury, or irritation of any of these nerves, or of the psoas, may cause pain at the top of your vulva.

There are also nerves on either side of the lower buttock that provide sensation to the skin of the buttocks and back part of the vulva—the inferior cluneal nerves. We have seen these be injured in sports and accidents, causing severe vulvar pain and sitting pain. Less commonly, the obturator nerves in the pelvis may be injured by surgery or orthopedic problems, especially related to the hip. Thinking outside the box helps detect these kinds of nerve problems, making them available for successful treatments.

Injury in the Central Nervous System

Any problem in your spinal cord might easily translate into sexual pain. We have seen some women whose deep pelvic pain, anal pain, or vaginal pain is due to bulging disks in their lumbosacral spine, causing stenosis (compression) of the spinal cord itself. Spinal-cord compression may also be associated with numbness, abnormal tingling, and sexual dysfunction. One of Deborah's patients lost her sexual sensation for seemingly mysterious reasons until she was finally found to have an old lower-back fracture from a fall she took many years earlier. The fracture had never been diagnosed, and over the years, it had steadily gotten worse, until compression and numbness ultimately resulted. Fortunately, surgery to repair the injury gradually allowed this woman's nerves to heal and her sexual function to resume. (As for pain that may worsen due to changes in the brain, our most important pain organ, see "The Central Nervous System" in Chapter 5.)

Disorders in the Autonomic Nervous System

Disorders in the autonomic nervous system also cause pain and affect our central experience of pain. When something goes wrong in our autonomic nervous system, our pelvic organs tend to suffer, especially the bladder and bowel. Due to the visceral–somatic reflex, in which nerves serving the organs and nerves serving the muscles get their signals crossed and affect one another (see "Cross-Talk: When Somatic and Visceral Pain Are Confused," in Chapter 5), the surrounding muscular and connective tissue structures become involved in the pain. As a result, both organs and muscles need to be treated in order to reduce this type of nerve pain (see Chapters 10 and 12).

Due in part to the visceral–somatic reflex, nerve pain commonly coexists with:

- painful bladder syndrome: Some 80 percent of women with nerve pain report more urgency and frequency of urination than normal and have a positive potassium test, which indicates chronic bladder inflammation.

- irritable bowel syndrome: Some 80 percent of women with nerve pain also have this condition.

DIAGNOSIS: THE TESTS YOU NEED

Chronic sexual pain is one of the most commonly misdiagnosed and mistreated conditions in all of medicine. We've seen dozens of patients whose doctors didn't perform the correct diagnostic tests to properly identify their disorders—or, in some cases, didn't perform any tests at all but instead relied on a quick look. This section is to help you ensure that your physician is ordering the right tests to create a good diagnosis and treatment plan. If he or she is not ordering these tests, you probably want to consider finding another doctor.

Bringing in an entire team is especially important with nerve pain. Specialists in neurology, orthopedics, physiatry, pain management, and physical therapy can often help diagnose the problem—and they can certainly help treat it. To attain overall healing, we also need to evaluate for what we call comorbidities: conditions that exist at the same time, such as painful bladder syndrome and irritable bowel syndrome (see Chapter 12).

Essential to a diagnosis is a good history, in which your doctor listens to your story from the beginning to detect just where your nerve pain might have begun. Hints that nerve pain has occurred are often easy to miss, but detecting "pain generators" can direct the rest of your evaluation. Likewise, during the physical exam, we want to get to the bottom of how this whole process may have gotten started, so that we can identify and individually treat anything that sets off your nerves. For example, perhaps a skin condition started the nerve pain; if it continues, it must be healed. If tight pelvic floor muscles are irritating the pudendal nerve, they must be identified and treated. See Chapter 5 to identify other potential causes of sexual pain.

If your physician suspects nerve pain, the next step is a neurological exam to determine the location and extent of the nerve disorder. Through touch and pressure, your physician should look for the following symptoms:

- numbness;

- allodynia (burning, sharp, or pin-prick pain from just a light touch);

- hyperalgesia (a mildly uncomfortable stimulus causes an unusual amount of pain); and/or

- reflex tests of pudendal-nerve function, such as the "bulbocaver-nosus reflex" and the "anal wink."

Where these symptoms occur tells us which nerves or branches may be involved. Your doctor's questions should help identify other potentially disordered nerves. Here are some clues:

- Pudendal-nerve pain usually makes sitting painful, except on a toilet.

- Ilioinguinal, iliohypogastric, and genitofemoral nerves don't usually cause seated pain but do often coexist with seemingly minor bulging disk problems between the vertebrae in the middle of your back.

- Spinal-cord pain such as from stenosis is worse with standing and walking, better with sitting.

Palpating for tenderness along your nerves can also reveal the source of the problem. For example, during a vaginal exam, touching the pudendal nerve with a finger at a prominent point on the inner pubic bone may elicit sharp, radiating pain if the pudendal nerve is involved. Tenderness at the upper rim of the pubic bone, at the course of the ilioinguinal nerve, may mean that that ilioinguinal nerve is inflamed.

Usually, the tests just described are enough to begin treatment. However, sometimes your doctor needs to run additional tests to rule out other problems.

Imaging is often useful, so your doctor may order an ultrasound, x-ray, MRI, or a CT scan (though we try to avoid that one, to reduce radiation exposure). MRIs are best and are technically improving for the soft-tissue pelvic floor structures, such as muscles and nerves. In our opinion, women with chronic sexual and vulvar pain have been neglected by the medical system until very recently, because they have not been considered for the up-to-date diagnostic imaging that is often quickly ordered for other pain conditions. In other medical fields—such as neurology, orthopedics, and ear, nose, and throat—a localized pain is investigated with imaging anytime there is a suspicion of a structural problem. Yet the bias toward sexual pain is that this cannot be a "structural" problem, going along with the "it's all in your head" myth. Deborah has to fight constantly with insurance companies with this mentality to get coverage for needed MRIs for our patients.

However, the situation is improving. Hollis Potter, MD—Chief of Magnetic Resonance Imaging at the Hospital for Special Surgery in New York City—has shown that, with correct technique and interpretation, much diagnostic help can come from imaging the pelvic floor with an MRI. We can obtain information about scarring in the fascia and other connective tissue around nerve branches, muscle and bony distortions, and tendon inflammation—which aids greatly in planning treatment. We hope that this technology and skill will soon be more widely available, and that the pelvic floor will be evaluated as it should be for all women with sexual pain.

There are also several types of nerve-function tests that may help us determine if one of your nerves is injured or malfunctioning. These tests are more difficult to perform on your pelvis as opposed to on your arms or legs, and as a result, many neurologists simply don't bother to check these areas when performing a neurological evaluation. We know that sounds shocking, but it's true—and it's another reason that you have to be more proactive than you ever dreamed when monitoring your own medical treatment. While we don't expect you to develop medical expertise in this area, we do think it's helpful for you to know all the tests that might be ordered, so that you can at least discuss them with your physician and find out what is and is not being done. If your doctor or specialist isn't performing any of the following tests and can't give you a good explanation as to why, you may want to look for more-informed care.

Special Nerve Function Tests

We still have lots to learn about the electrical and chemical behavior of our nerves in their role as information movers. In some situations, it may be valuable for you to have one of the special tests below to find out more about why you have nerve pain.

AUTONOMIC-NERVE STUDIES FOR SMALL FIBERS

Small fibers are the thinnest strands running within your nerves. Some of them carry pain signals, others transmit other types of sensation, and most are part of the autonomic nervous system.

These tests look at small-fiber function and anatomy with the idea that if autonomic nerves are abnormal, then pain fibers probably are too. Your small fibers are tested indirectly in a number of different ways (without needles), including checking blood pressure and pulse changes on a tilt table and evaluating temperature and sweat-gland function. Occasionally, in very confusing cases, we may also perform a tiny skin biopsy to stain specifically for these small nerve fibers. When they have been damaged they have abnormal shapes and are present in much lower numbers. Documenting this physical disorder helps us decide on systemic pain medications and surgical procedures, and many of our patients feel that it lessens some of the frustration of not knowing what's wrong.

PERIPHERAL-NERVE STUDIES

In the following three tests, surface electrodes (tiny needles) are used to stimulate the nerves or muscles, and the response is measured.

- nerve-conduction studies, which can detect alterations in the speed of sensory or pain impulses common in nerve diseases;

- electromyography (EMG), which tests motor-nerve root function; and

- somatosensory evoked-potential studies, which check to make sure that nerves are properly delivering signals to the spinal cord, and which help to detect any pinched nerves.

INJECTIONS OF NUMBING AGENTS

Injections may be given to find out whether a numbing agent applied to a particular nerve gives pain relief, allowing us to identify which nerves are causing the pain.

Systemic Tests

Blood tests may be given for conditions that may predispose someone to nerve pain, and for conditions that may worsen it. The following are some conditions that may do this:

- diabetes;

- tick-associated infections such as Lyme disease;

- low levels of iron, zinc, vitamin D, and B vitamins;

- high levels of mercury or lead;

- digestive disorders such as gluten sensitivity and other nutritional deficiencies; and

- rheumatoid disorders and other autoimmune conditions.

TREATMENTS: WHAT YOU CAN EXPECT

The treatments described in this chapter will work to heal nerve pain—that's the good news. The bad news is that they may take a very long time—from three to six months in some cases, and up to a year or more in others. It's also possible that your physician and his or her team will have to experiment—with different treatments, with various diagnostic tools, and/or with different types of physical therapy.

However, there is a light at the end of the tunnel. There is every reason to believe you can reprogram your nerves to stop transmitting pain messages, and that you can reclaim your sex life—and your overall life—once more. Nerve pain requires more patience than the other types of pain in this book, but you have every reason to believe your patience will be rewarded.

When Deborah was in medical school, injured nerves were considered to be, by and large, beyond repair. What we've fortunately learned since then is that nerves are not untreatable—they simply heal very slowly. Research over the past three decades has shown that, without a doubt, nerves can heal, recover, reproduce, and regenerate. This knowledge has led to wonderful advances in therapy for patients formerly considered beyond help—including stroke victims with brain injury, people who have gone through an accidental amputation, and women who suffer from sexual pain. What we've learned is that it isn't only the severity of the trauma that counts, but also, how each person's body responds to the pain. Research into ways of altering the body's response to pain is ongoing—and is giving hope to all of us.

Overall Treatment Goals

No matter which type of nerve pain you have or where the pain-causing nerve is located, there are several general therapies you need that will get you started on the road to recovery.

- Remove any type of compression on the nerve. Restrict sitting, for instance, if it causes you pudendal-nerve pain.

- Ensure a good blood supply to the nerve (massage, physical therapy, yoga, tai chi, and qigong can all be helpful here).

- Get adequate oxygenation, through deep breathing and/or aerobic exercise.

- Get adequate sleep, allowing the body to heal.

- Reduce stress, which causes an increase in muscle tension, adding to nerve compression, and which also alters the body's chemistry and increases inflammation, worsening nerve damage.

- Get good nutrition to nourish injured nerves (see "Nourish your nerves and your body" in Chapter 4 for information on special nerve nutrients).

- Engage in a mind–body practice such as meditation, which has proven successful with all types of long-term chronic pain.

Noninvasive or Minimally Invasive Treatments

The number and types of treatments for nerve problems causing painful sex are rapidly expanding, and most women do not need invasive therapies like surgery in order to get better.

TOPICAL ANESTHETICS

Lidocaine, bupivacaine, and other topical anesthetics—often used in patch form—are helpful. We now also have a capsaicin patch. Capsaicin is the active component in hot peppers, and it desensitizes nerve endings for a period of time. Capsaicin patches can be applied for an hour in the doctor's office, and pain relief may last for three months.

TOPICAL "NERVE SEDATORS"

Topical medications that Deborah calls "nerve sedators" may also bring relief. These are compounded versions of medications that are usually taken orally, such as the many discussed in the Oral Pain Relievers section later in this chapter, and are applied as a cream or oil over the area of the disordered nerve. In this way we can deliver the medication to the involved area and usually avoid the side effects that they cause when ingested by mouth.

PHYSICAL THERAPY

This is a mainstay of treating nerve pain, as it can help by:

- releasing fascia and other soft-tissue tension around a restricted nerve;

- improving elasticity surrounding nerve tissues;

- increasing blood supply to the nerves;

- reversing muscle imbalance, which causes muscles to "behave inappropriately" and pull on nerves; and

- correcting movement and gait disorders, which may cause nerve pressure or traction.

INJECTIONS

Anesthetic and/or anti-inflammatory medications injected into the tissues surrounding the injured nerve (these are called "perineural injections") can be very helpful. So can trigger-point injections, which are administered to surrounding muscles that may be pinching nerves. Pelvic nerves that are amenable to such treatments include the following:

- the autonomic nerves surrounding the coccyx in the sympathetic plexus;

- the pudendal nerve, as it nears the sit bones, within the vagina, or in the lower back;

- the ilioinguinal, iliohypogastric, and genitofemoral nerves; and

- spinal nerve roots at the lumbosacral spine.

ACUPUNCTURE

This has also been helpful in treating chronic pain, including sexual pain.

OTHER LOCAL THERAPIES

The following may be helpful as well:

- transcutaneous electrical nerve stimulation devices (TENS units);

- pulsed radiofrequency nerve ablation, which involves inserting a small probe to temporarily stun the pudendal nerves or nerve roots;

- epidural steroid injections; and

- botulinum toxin A (Botox) administered to overactive muscles surrounding the nerve, which releases pressure on the nerve for up to three months, and which may have some direct effect on the irritated nerve itself.

ORAL PAIN RELIEVERS

Oral prescription medications have shown good evidence of success with nerve pain, as they calm both the injured nerve and the central nervous system itself. Many of these are often effective, including the following:

Oral Analgesics

Acetaminophen and nonsteroidal anti-inflammatory drugs (NSAIDs) are useful and relatively safe pain reducers.

Anticonvulsants

These probably work at several levels along the neuropathways to reduce pain; examples are gabapentin (Neurontin), pregabalin (Lyrica), and topiramide (Topamax).

Antidepressants

Most selective serotonin reuptake inhibitors (SSRIs) are not effective in treating nerve pain. However, other types of antidepressants do have pain-relief properties. These include tricyclics such as amitriptyline (Elavil) and nortriptyline (Pamelor), and serotonin–norepinephrine reuptake inhibitors (SNRIs), such as duloxetine (Cymbalta), milnacipran (Savella), and venlafaxine (Effexor).

Other Medications

There are some other options as well. Anti-arrhythmic medications such as mexiletine behave like lidocaine in quieting the nerves.

Muscle relaxants can be useful if overly excitable muscles are squeezing the nerve (see Chapter 10).

One class of medications that is currently in clinical trials is NMDA (N-methyl-D-aspartate) inhibitors, which seem to prevent acute pain from progressing into neuropathic pain. So far we've seen many side effects with ketamine, but fewer with the milder medications such as amantadine and memantidine.

Opioid-like medications such as tramadol (Ultram) and tapentadol (Nucynta) have of late been found to soothe the brain changes that may occur with chronic pain, and also benefit the neurotransmitters to decrease pain.

BE CAREFUL WITH OPIOIDS!

Opioids may be useful for some types of nerve pain but should be taken only with careful consideration and with close monitoring by your physician. See the boxed text, "Avoid Opioid Pain Medications," in Chapter 5 for more information on the potential benefits of opioids.

Surgical Treatments

If noninvasive therapies are not effective, and if it is ascertained that a nerve is being compressed by surrounding bone, a spinal disk, a ligament, inelastic fibrous tissue, or anatomical "tunnels," surgery may prove effective. Surgery may release larger nerves (including the pudendal nerve), peripheral nerves, and nerve branches. Since recuperation may be prolonged, however, easier therapies should be tried first.

NEUROLYSIS

Pudendal-nerve decompression surgery, also called neurolysis, is the breaking up or release of adhesions that pull on, squeeze, or stretch a nerve. In addition, neurolysis sometimes involves removing the damaged portion of the nerve itself. In other cases, ligaments around the nerve are cut, giving the nerve more freedom. We don't really know what the overall success rate is, because the procedure is done differently by different specialists on different kinds of problems. But many doctors are getting together to work on this and find out which women would be the best candidates. We are also following up on those women who, as part of the surgery, undergo incision of their sacrotuberous ligament to free the pudendal nerve, since historically there has been a concern about this causing instability of the sacroiliac joint. So far, for women who have been correctly diagnosed, the outcome seems to be good. Of course, it is critical that you seek the care of the most skilled nerve surgeon in your area—one with good experience in operating on small peripheral nerves. (For more information on this procedure see the Resources section for the book *Pain Solutions,* which can be downloaded for free.)

NEUROMODULATION

Also known as "spinal-cord stimulation," this is a technique that strives to affect the neuropathway and function of nerves close to the spinal cord. The spinal cord is the gateway that forwards sensations of pain to the brain, so this technique attempts to modify and partially close the gate. Local spinal-cord chemistry seems to be affected, which also reduces pain-signal transmission.

In this outpatient procedure, a weeklong trial is conducted first: A wire lead is inserted into one of the openings of the sacrum containing a nerve root. Electrical impulses go through the lead to realign or even "scramble" the nerve impulses that carry the pain messages to the spine and then to the brain. If this preliminary procedure is successful, the permanent lead is placed, and through a small incision, a generator battery is implanted under the skin of the abdomen or buttocks. An external "remote control" is used to adjust the electrical stimulation from that point on. Thousands of people with chronic-pain syndromes have done well with this technique over the past forty years, and the technology continues to improve.

PAIN PUMPS

Medications (usually opioids) can be administered through permanently implanted epidural or spinal catheters, blocking the transmission of pain impulses going up the pathway to the brain.

HOW *NOT* TO TREAT NERVE PAIN

Do *not* . . .

- delay treatment: Time is of the essence, since the longer the nerves continue to transmit the pain, the more prone they are to malfunction.

- give up hope: Nerve pain is complicated, but there are lots of treatments currently available—and there are more in the research pipeline.

POTENTIAL BREAKTHROUGHS: LOOKING TOWARD THE FUTURE

Several very promising techniques are being researched. Hyperbaric oxygen—which is basically oxygen under pressure—seems to increase oxygen in the blood flow to damaged nerves, potentially speeding their healing. Smaller and even portable machines are now available, making this option possible for more women.

Another promising area involves working at the spinal-cord level with new medications to affect the nerve messages carried through the spine up to the brain. We're also optimistic about improvements in energy technology (like pulsed radiofrequency), which is used to reprogram pain processing in the spinal cord.

Finally, brain magnetic stimulation—in which magnets are used to stimulate areas in the brain—and transcranial direct-current stimulation—in which electricity is likewise used—both seem very promising for chronic severe pain. We are aware of at least one stubborn case of chronic vulvar pain that responded remarkably to this type of treatment.

Meanwhile, the women we treat who struggle with nerve pain develop deep inner resources to deal with their condition.

For Sandra, religious faith is the key. When things get bad, she watches a religious program on television or reminds herself that God has a purpose for her life.

Lynn's mainstay is her support system. "A few weeks ago, we were in a restaurant, and I went over to say hello to a bunch of people I knew sitting at another table," she says. "One of the husbands came over to me and asked, 'How's your vagina?' I said, 'The same,' and that ended that. I didn't get embarrassed. He wasn't teasing me; he was concerned and felt comfortable enough to ask me straight out. I find this kind of support very reassuring and helpful." In addition, Lynn says, "My sense of humor keeps me going. When I lose that, I know I am depressed. I regain it by talking to my husband, my sister, or my friends, or I go out to dinner. I also know that so much research is now being done, and I have to believe that there will be something soon that may not cure me but will help ease my pain."

10

PELVIC FLOOR PAIN

Until three years ago, I had great, orgasmic, fulfilling sex. And then I noticed I started to feel irritation during intercourse. Initially, I didn't have pain upon penetration, but the longer he was in me, the more irritated I would become. I also began to develop urinary frequency—once or twice an hour and four times at night. As time went on, my vagina became very sore. The pain felt like it was emanating from my vagina and urethra. The irritation grew in intensity and length, to the point that my pain level reached 7 or 8 out of 10.

—BLAIR, A TEACHER IN HER FIFTIES

I first noticed that sex was painful right after my boyfriend moved in with me two years ago. We had been having a normal sex life until then, and suddenly, sexual intercourse became painful. And I noticed I couldn't even put a tampon in without screaming in pain. But we still continued to have sex, and I would just grin and bear it. I never thought it was a psychological thing, but I knew it was going to hurt when we tried to have intercourse, and I would crunch up and make it a million times worse. Eventually the pain was so bad that we couldn't have intercourse anymore.

—LUCY, FASHION MAGAZINE EDITOR, AGE TWENTY-SEVEN

PELVIC FLOOR PAIN: AN OVERVIEW

You can't tell exactly where the pain is coming from—it just hurts. Sometimes you can feel your muscles spasm. Sometimes you just feel sore. You might feel something pressing on your bladder, which makes you keep running to the bathroom, or feeling as though you always have to go. It's all so painful; you can't stand to be touched; and you certainly can't imagine having sex.

Although your vulva and vagina are not the source of the pain, you feel pain there—and perhaps also in the muscles around your anal opening and rectum. The muscle pressure may even cause you to develop anal fissures, as your muscles thicken, and shorten, and press. Yet when you go to a doctor, you hear that you just need to relax, or maybe even that your problems stem from tension and anxiety around sex. You know there's something really wrong—that the problem is not just "in your head." But you've been told that so many times that it is, and now you're beginning to wonder. . . .

Well, let us put your mind at ease. Your problem is not in your head. You're suffering from pelvic floor dysfunction—a problem with the muscles that support your entire pelvic region. Because this area of our bodies can't be easily seen, even with an x-ray (though some aspects may be inferred from those images), the importance of the pelvic floor muscles has never been appreciated by modern medicine until very recently. Finally, though, we're beginning to recognize the crucial role this region plays in our anatomy, bodily functions, and sexual experience.

Disorders in this region are definitely treatable, and you can look forward to a full recovery—though you may have to make a lifelong commitment to getting proper exercise and physical therapy. Since pelvic floor disorders are involved in sexual function and in so many types of sexual pain, caring for that region of your body is a terrific investment in lifelong sexual health.

SYMPTOMS OF PELVIC FLOOR CONDITIONS

If you are suffering from pelvic floor pain, you are likely to have one or more of the following symptoms:

- muscle spasms and sensations of aching, burning, and tightness in the genital area (made worse by sitting);

- during or after intercourse, pain at the vaginal opening or deeper in the vaginal canal;

- cramping and throbbing pain when touched in the pelvic region; or

- pain that worsens as the day goes on, and that is worst at bedtime.

HOW PELVIC FLOOR DYSFUNCTION AFFECTS YOU

Anything that creates an imbalance in the muscles and fascia of the pelvic floor can create sexual pain. The following are some causes of such an imbalance:

- a congenital or hereditary tendency to either high muscle tension (also known as "high-tone problems") or low muscle tension (which means that your pelvic muscles aren't properly supporting the organs in your pelvis);

- a congenitally small or short bony pelvis and/or pelvic floor;

- physiologically "normal" hypermobility of joints, ligaments, and fascia within the pelvic floor, part of our design for pregnancy and delivery;

- neurologic conditions (such as myasthenia gravis and cerebral palsy) that affect muscle tone;

- congenital orthopedic issues (such as developmental hip dysplasia) that imbalance the pelvic floor muscles;

- injuries to the pelvic floor (often caused by childbirth or auto accidents);

- back injuries that make the pelvic floor compensate for poor back strength;

- trauma to the coccyx or pubic bone (as can easily happen in sports or from falls);

- repetitive strain from some sports and exercises (such as biking, gymnastics, competitive cheerleading, skiing, or ballet—all of which require the pelvic floor muscles to be held in contraction for long periods of time);

- a "tensing-up" reflex response to other causes of sexual pain, such as vestibulodynia and endometriosis;

- irritable bowel syndrome, and repeated straining from constipation or tightening with diarrhea;

- painful bladder syndrome or overactive bladder, as the muscles respond to frequent urination;

- a "tensing-up" response to a painful sexual injury, a vaginal or pelvic infection, or a urinary tract infection;

- an autoimmune condition that affects the normal function of muscles; or

- fibromyalgia.

Although we're learning more all the time (for example, the recognition of orthopedic or autoimmune influences on the pelvic floor is quite recent), we still have a lot to learn. Consequently, for many women, it can be difficult for doctors to identify a particular trigger. We can be sure, however, that if the pelvic floor muscles are imbalanced, sexual pain is likely to follow.

So what happens when these muscles are injured or abnormal? Generally, we see a wide range of maladies, and any woman might have one or several—including areas of inappropriate tightening and shortening, trigger points, tense bands of muscles, and reflexive muscle gripping. With injury may also come an overgrowth (or "thickening") of the supportive fascia and other connective tissue, which in turn further restricts the muscles. Elastic tissues lose their flexibility in a process we call "fibrosis."

Tendons may scar and consequently lose some of their flexibility as well. Tendons connect muscle to bone, so they're an especially sensitive area that can quickly reflect—or cause—muscular distress. A condition known as tendinosis frequently occurs after inflammation—which, as we have seen, is often associated with heat, redness, pain, and swelling. Even when the inflammation subsides and the swelling goes away, pain might continue, due to the scarring that the tendon developed during the inflammatory episode. The scarring further acts to decrease blood supply, and the whole process leads the body to produce new inflammatory chemicals. As a result, the tendon becomes dry, ischemic (a term used to describe the results of low blood supply), and prone to further injury. This degeneration of the tendons' connective tissue fibers can now be seen better than ever on Magnetic Resonance Imaging. We also know now that physical therapy can help alleviate this condition.

Injuries to the tendons can thus have far-reaching effects. Even after injuries have healed, MRIs reveal that the scarring remains—perhaps also with an ongoing restriction of blood supply and other ill effects. Tendinosis, scarring, and other results of the muscles' imbalance also often cause or result in inflammation, compression, and/or entrapment of the pudendal and other pelvic nerves—all of which worsen sexual pain.

As we mentioned in Chapter 8, women who are unable to have sex because of vaginal clenching—or who can have sex only with enormous pain—have frequently been given the pseudoscientific diagnosis of "vaginismus." A number of muscle studies, including electromyography (EMG), have revealed what's really going on. Women diagnosed with vaginismus have pelvic floor muscles with "high tone," meaning that their muscles are always at least partially contracted—even at rest, and even when they aren't being touched. In addition, something as apparently minor as a stressful thought caused these women to unconsciously clench their pelvic floor—much as some people grind their teeth under stress. Some women also have hyperexcitable bulbocavernosus muscles (muscles right underneath the labia, as seen in illustration 10-2).

For these women, even a gentle touch in the pelvic region can provoke a quick, intense contraction of one or more muscles in the area. The tension can itself cause pain, and it can also contribute to an imbalance in the region. Pretty soon, other muscles are compensating for the tense weak ones, creating new sources of muscle tension and new imbalances. It's a painful, self-reinforcing vicious circle: Muscle tension, imbalance, inflammation, and tendinosis create more muscle tension, imbalance, inflammation, and tendinosis. And pain in the vulva, vagina, and rectum is the result.

What is causing your muscles to react so swiftly and extremely? We're not entirely sure, especially because many causes may be involved. Certainly, you might be suffering from a malfunctioning central nervous system. You might have been born with or have developed a specific muscle tone that is more vulnerable to this type of imbalance. We're often not sure whether the nerve abnormality or the muscle tension comes first in this disorder, but we do know that both are often present, and that each needs to be addressed.

Another underlying cause of pelvic floor dysfunction is other types of sexual pain, since the pelvic floor muscles tend to tense reflexively in response to pain in the vaginal opening or the vulvar region. If you're experiencing enough sexual pain, your muscles may "learn" to remain tense and tightly contracted. The more they tense, the shorter they become, and the less they allow penetration.

As you can see, pelvic floor dysfunction can be caused by many factors—and each of those factors can trigger any or all of the others. Meanwhile, this dysfunction can affect your life in a variety of ways. Daily and/or unprovoked achiness interferes with sitting, biking, stretching, and other activities. Imbalanced muscles often press on the urethra and the base of the bladder, creating a constant urge to urinate that worsens with sexual activity. Perianal muscles are often involved, causing painful defecation, constipation, and often very painful anal fissures. The pain worsens as the day goes on and as your muscles tire, so that you feel best after a good night's sleep and worst at bedtime.

THE EMOTIONAL SIDE EFFECTS OF SEXUAL PAIN

Besides the physical effects of pelvic floor dysfunction, there are psychological, emotional, and "daily life" effects that create pain of their own.

In the past, Blair couldn't sit in a car for longer than fifteen minutes at a time. "My parents live about an hour and a half away, and I couldn't visit them. I felt horrible about that. But if I sat in the car for fifteen minutes, it became so painful, and I would pay for it for at least two days later," she says. "I felt like the pain was taking my life force from me." She was also depleted by the frequent anxiety attacks she experienced whenever her pain flared up. "I could deal with a painful flare-up when it lasted for a short time," she says, "but when it went on for a few days, my anxiety level went through the roof. Thankfully, although I still have some pain, because of all the treatment I have received, especially my physical therapy, I can go on long car rides and I experience very little anxiety."

>

> The effects of Lucy's pelvic floor dysfunction went to the very core of her womanhood. "I understand why women often feel less feminine when they lose their breasts," she says. "Your vagina also makes you feel like a woman, and when that doesn't work, you don't feel like a real woman anymore. I could use that part of my body to go to the bathroom, but that was its only purpose at that point."

Lucy ultimately improved remarkably in her pelvic floor pain with physical therapy. This form of sexual pain has one of the best prognoses of all.

WHAT'S GOING ON: THE BIOLOGY

The pelvic floor is a bowl-like area within the core of your body. It's located right between your pelvic bones—your pubic bones at your front and sides, and your tailbone and sacrum at the base of your spine. This crucial area is composed of strong interconnected muscles, tendons, ligaments, and connective tissue that hold the bones of the pelvis together.

Within every woman's pelvis sit three separate organ systems: reproductive, gastrointestinal, and urinary. Your pelvic floor supports these organs, as well as your spine and the entire core of your body. As if that weren't enough work for one body region to do, your pelvic floor also contains muscles that connect your legs to your core, participating in your gait and balance.

We hope you're beginning to appreciate this extraordinary central region of your body, and that you're starting to understand how a muscular disorder here could have such a painful impact on so many of your systems.

How is this region involved in sexual pain? Within your pelvic floor, a complicated weave of several muscles surrounds your vaginal canal. These muscles and tissues are directly involved in your sexual pleasure and in your experience of orgasm. Many of the erectile tissues in the lower vagina that add to arousal and orgasm are intimately supported by the pelvic floor muscles, so spasms in those muscles not only cause decreased blood flow but also interfere with your sexual responses. If something goes wrong here, it's going to have an immediate, direct, and painful effect on your sex life.

Specifically, if the muscles of your pelvic floor malfunction, you'll begin to feel tightness and/or spasms—which you are likely to experience not as muscle distress but as severe pain in your vulvar, vaginal, or pelvic organ regions, and possibly around your anus and rectum.

Women seem to be more at risk for pelvic floor problems than men, although many men also suffer from this condition. Due to our female anatomy and childbearing design, our pelvis is broader and shallower, requiring more muscle strength and connective tissue stiffness for stability. Our hormones affect these tissues and contribute to excess flexibility and increased risk of injury. Studies estimate that anywhere between 4 and 24 percent of women currently suffer from pelvic floor pain. (The wide range of this statistic makes it clear how much we need more research.)

The Specific Muscles Involved

Pelvic floor dysfunction can take a wide variety of forms, depending on which muscles are most affected. Refer to illustrations 10-1 and 10-2 as you read further to understand the location and attachments of the many pelvic floor muscles. When any one of these muscles goes out of balance, shortens, or remains clenched, the resulting pain can be "referred" throughout the entire region, so that you feel it in a variety of places that seem far from its actual source.

We have found that it's helpful for women with sexual pain to be able to visualize exactly what's going on, so we've provided some "likely suspects" for muscles that might be involved in your pelvic floor dysfunction. Any or all of the muscle groups listed on page 214 might be involved, and you may or may not be able to relate your "lived experience" of pain to its actual source. But this list should at least help you begin the process of visualizing your pelvic region, so that you can start to understand the pain you feel.

Illustration 10-1.

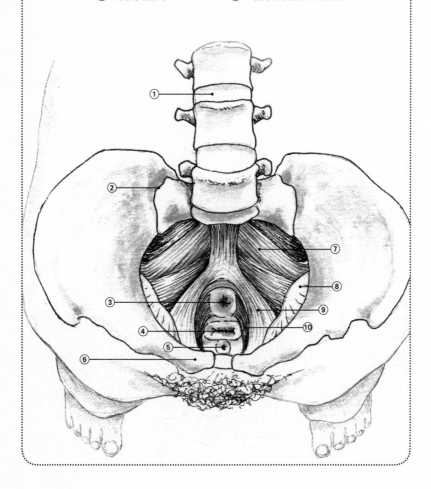

DEEP PELVIC FLOOR

1. Lumbar Spine
2. Sacroiliac Joint
3. Rectum
4. Vagina
5. Urethra
6. Pubic Bone
7. Iliococcygeus Muscle
8. Obturator Internus Muscle
9. Pubococcygeus Muscle
10. Puborectalis Muscle

Illustration 10-2.

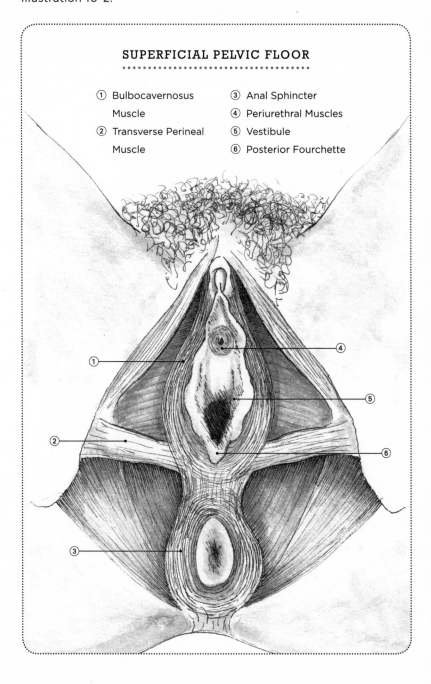

SUPERFICIAL PELVIC FLOOR

① Bulbocavernosus Muscle

② Transverse Perineal Muscle

③ Anal Sphincter

④ Periurethral Muscles

⑤ Vestibule

⑥ Posterior Fourchette

Muscles at the vaginal opening include the bulbocavernosus, puborecta-lis, and transverse perineal, as shown in illustrations 10-1 and 10-2. If these muscles are malfunctioning, penetration may be quite painful.

Muscles around the bladder and urethra include the puborectalis and pubococcygeus. In this case, you are likely to feel pressure in your bladder—and you either to have to urinate frequently, or feel like you do. You may also have painful bladder syndrome, which can in turn cause other types of sexual pain. See illustration 12-1 in Chapter 12 for this muscle anatomy as it relates to the bladder.

Muscles around the rectum include the puborectalis, pubococcygeus, iliococcygeus, and anal sphincter. These are the muscles whose dysfunction leads to anal fissures, soreness in the rectum, and pain and bleeding when defecating.

Muscles to the side include the obturator internus and the pubococ-cygeus, and may compress the pudendal nerve. If these muscles are malfunc-tioning, you'll feel intense vaginal and/or vulvar pain, depending on where the pudendal nerve is compressed.

Muscles close to the hip and low back include the iliopsoas muscles and conjoined tendon, the piriformis muscles, and the gluteal muscles (in your buttocks). Problems here may feel like lower-back or hip pain, or may cause pain that radiates to your vulva or rectum. Illustrations 11-1 and 11-2 in Chapter 11 will help you understand this part of the anatomy.

Muscles close to the front (anterior) abdominal wall and upper pelvis include the iliopsoas muscles and tendon, the rectus abdominus, and the internal and external obliques. Injuries, scars, or tension in these muscles may radiate pain to the clitoris or masquerade as pelvic organ pain and be misdiagnosed as endometriosis.

Another advantage of identifying the muscles that are malfunctioning is that you can then treat them with self-massage, and can work with a physi-cal therapist to strengthen them. This kind of work can be going on while you are waiting for your physician's treatment to take effect—or even while you are seeking the right physician.

COMMON MISDIAGNOSES
FOR PELVIC FLOOR DYSFUNCTION

MISDIAGNOSIS	HOW TO RULE IT OUT
Recurrent bladder/urethra infection	Specific bacterial cultures
Painful bladder syndrome	Often coexist; cystoscopy
Vaginismus	Pelvic floor exam
Overactive bladder syndrome	Symptoms persist after treatment
Endometriosis	Pelvic exam, imaging studies, laparoscopy
Ovarian cysts	Pelvic exam, ultrasound
Lumbar spine disc disease	Physical exam, imaging studies, nerve studies
Psychological illness	MD awareness/education

DIAGNOSIS: THE TESTS YOU NEED

Chronic sexual pain is one of the most commonly misdiagnosed and mistreated conditions in all of medicine. We've seen dozens of patients whose doctors didn't perform the correct diagnostic tests to properly identify their disorders—or, in some cases, didn't perform any tests at all but instead relied on a quick look. This section is to help you ensure that your physician is ordering the right tests to create a good diagnosis and treatment plan. If he or she is not ordering these tests, you probably want to consider finding another doctor.

As always, the first, essential step is a good clinical examination, which is the mainstay of your doctor's diagnosis. Your doctor should look closely at your vulvar region, where asymmetry in the structures of your vulva may reflect underlying muscles pulling in an imbalanced direction. Touching the skin of your vulva can also cause any hyperexcitable muscles to tense and clench reflexively—often so dramatically that your doctor can actually see the reaction. In particular, your doctor should evaluate your bulbocaverno-sus muscles this way.

You should also be given a digital ("finger") vaginal and rectal exam, in which the doctor gently touches you with one finger in an organized way, proceeding through all areas of the pelvic floor. Your doctor is feeling for tight muscle bands, tender spots, fibrous or nonelastic fascia, and muscle weakness. He or she is also looking for bone abnormalities, including check-ing to see if structures such as your ischial spines (the prominent areas of your inner pubic bone, near the pudendal nerves) or pubic arch (the lower edge of your pubic bone) are abnormally shaped or sized. Your doctor should also be feeling for asymmetry in muscles from left to right, tenderness in the coccyx, tenderness to touch in the obturator internus muscle, and ten-derness in response to hip flexion or rotation. Finally, a digital exam should explore anal-sphincter tone and tension, and also identify whether you have anal fissures or hemorrhoids.

In some cases, your doctor might need to take advantage of new imag-ing techniques that give us a window into the world of the pelvic floor. A dedicated high-resolution pelvic floor MRI might show pelvic floor injuries that are difficult to ascertain with just a visual or digital exam. For example, an MRI scan might pick up:

- tendinosis;

- muscle atrophy or hypertrophy;

- nerve compression;

- pubic-bone inflammation;

- fractures or a significant deviation of the coccyx; and/or

- abnormal vasculature and/or varicosities (swollen, enlarged veins).

Your doctor may also order blood tests looking for rare diseases, vitamin deficiencies, or infections such as Lyme disease—any of which can affect your muscle health.

Meanwhile, another essential component of your diagnosis is an expert exam by a physical therapist to evaluate your pelvic floor. We can't stress this too strongly. Treatment of sexual pain is a team effort, and if any member of the team is missing, the patient is the one who suffers.

TREATMENTS: WHAT YOU CAN EXPECT

The very good news is that pelvic floor dysfunction is treatable—more easily so than many other types of sexual pain. The sooner you can get treatment, the better, so that the nerves running through your pelvis are not restricted or compressed by malfunctioning muscles, which might lead to nerve irritation and then neuropathic pain. If we catch pelvic floor dysfunction late, we have to deal with a range of muscle, nerve, and biochemical issues, so treatment is likely to be longer and more complicated. Success is possible, however—especially if you are committed to physical therapy and the self-care regimes that can make a difference.

First, make sure you're taking good care of yourself. Ensure the best sleep you can, so your pelvic floor muscles can rest. You should also be sure to regulate your bowel movements to avoid constipation and straining, which affect your pelvic floor muscles. Adding fiber to your diet and making other dietary changes can help right away. So can additional exercise. But if you have an underlying systemic muscle dysfunction, your treatment should also be focused on healing that.

Warm baths can be soothing when pain flares up. Some oral medications may also be useful, such as NSAIDs (nonsteroidal anti-inflammatory drugs, such as aspirin and ibuprofen) and oral or topical muscle relaxants. (If your physician has identified nerve pain as a component of your condition, see Oral Pain Relievers section in Chapter 9, for other beneficial medications.)

There are a lot of alternative healing modalities that can help muscle pain. Consider Bikram yoga, which is conducted in an extremely warm environment that relaxes and softens your muscles. Certain supplements are also good for muscle nutrition (see the boxed text "Feed Your Muscles").

PREPARING FOR A PELVIC FLOOR PHYSICAL THERAPIST

A physical therapist who is knowledgeable and trained in helping sexual-pain patients will often do an internal exam. This is surprising to some women. Niva Herzig, PT, MPT, BCB-PMD, often sees this surprise with new patients.

"When patients come to my office," she says, "they look at me in shock when I say I am going to do an internal exam. They are stunned when I ask them to remove their pants and underwear."

Sometimes they are so uncomfortable that she realizes it's better to give them time. "When I see someone is not ready for an internal exam, or to remove their clothes or have their genitals examined, I will not pursue this avenue but will show them a picture of the anatomy, and I show them the relationship of the muscles, and how I can assess those muscles."

Then she lets her patients sit with the information. "Usually when these patients leave and go home, they begin to understand the process, and they start to get over their embarrassment. Usually after a couple of weeks, they begin to feel safe."

Physical Therapy

Your mainstay here, again, is physical therapy. We don't know everything about how these manual and muscle techniques work, though we believe they improve blood flow, rid the muscles of toxic chemicals (like lactic acid) that have built up as a result of ischemia, and improve muscle activity—which in turn reduces inflammation. Even though we don't know exactly *how* these techniques work, we know that they absolutely *do* work.

We're always distressed when our patients are resistant to or casual about their physical therapy—much as we would be if a diabetic wasn't taking her insulin on schedule, or if a heart patient kept eating fried foods. Yes, it can be hard to commit to an exercise regime—especially if you're busy and overwhelmed with work and life. We understand—both of us are working mothers, and we frequently feel overwhelmed as well. But physical therapy is absolutely crucial to recovery from pelvic floor dysfunction. Without it, your prognosis is dim. With it, you have a wonderful prospect of full recovery, which you can maintain as long as you continue to exercise.

Even though it can be hard to regularly follow a physical therapist's suggested exercises, we suggest that you make a list of all the reasons you might want to stick to this regime. Then ask yourself what your priorities are. Chances are, you'll see that the benefits of sticking to the regime are well worth the time and effort.

Specialized physical therapy techniques will help you:

- increase blood flow to restricted muscles and fascia of the pelvic floor;

- increase muscle elasticity;

- lengthen chronically contracted muscles;

- improve muscle strength;

- mobilize scarred fascia, ligaments, and tendons;

- move restricting tissues off nerve branches;

- rebalance muscles, so that they all are participating in your core stability in a coordinated way;

- rehabilitate your anal sphincter muscles and the base of your bladder; and

- strengthen your hip rotators and your back and abdominal muscles so that your pelvic floor doesn't have to compensate for them.

FEED YOUR MUSCLES

These nutrients are good for combating pelvic floor dysfunction. They are either needed "food" for muscles to use to grow and maintain themselves, or supplements that may help muscle function, and are available over the counter.

- magnesium malate or citrate, 400mg daily;

- vitamin D3, 2000 i.u. daily;

- omega-3 fatty-acid supplements, 1000 to 2000mg a day, in addition to a diet high in flaxseed and fish oils;

- gamma-linolenic acid supplements, 500mg daily max (found in borage seed oil, black currant seed oil, evening primrose oil);

- SAM-e, going slowly up from 100mg to 400mg daily, in two or three divided doses; and

- methylsulfonylmethane (MSM), 500mg a day, and matched with the same amount of vitamin C. Do not use this product if you are allergic to sulfa.

You can also benefit from estrogens in the form of compounded estradiol or estriol, used intravaginally to increase blood flow to muscles. These are prescribed by your doctor and made by special compounding pharmacists.

Muscle Relaxers

In some cases, trigger-point injections into the tense or tender muscle areas can help the muscles relax. The placement of diazepam (Valium), a muscle relaxant, into the vagina for a course of therapy, or to help flares, can be quite useful. As a tablet, as a compounded suppository, or as a gel, the diazepam is only minimally absorbed into your system, so you're unlikely to feel anything except local muscle relaxation.

Botulinum toxin A (Botox) injections into high-tone, contracted, pelvic floor muscles can also be very effective. They are no substitute for physical therapy, and they should never be relied upon as your primary treatment—but if you need help in getting specific muscle areas to relax, Botox can help keep the areas looser for up to three months. If you rely on it for the long term, however, Botox can actually be detrimental. Because the "Botoxed" muscles are not being used, they become weaker, setting you up for further problems down the road. So use it cautiously—but generally speaking, it's very safe.

Vaginal Dilators

You should also begin using a vaginal dilator to help open your vaginal canal and work the muscles in that region. You may do this with or without the guidance of a doctor or physical therapist. Here are the steps for using dilators, which come as a set of various sizes.

1. Find a private place.

2. Use a lubricant of your choice (for suggestions see the Chapter 14 boxed text "Lubricants Are Our Friends"), and cover the smallest dilator with it.

3. Consciously relax your thighs, buttocks, and abdomen.

4. Slide the dilator into your vagina until it is about halfway in, pausing if you notice any tightening, burning, or other discomfort.

5. To release tension, visualize your vagina and pelvic floor as soft, stretchy, and relaxed. Breathe deeply, allowing yourself to release your muscles with every exhalation. Make sure you soften your belly and leave your legs limp.

6. If possible, leave the dilator inside your vagina for fifteen minutes at a time while resting comfortably.

Perform this exercise each day, gradually progressing to a wider dilator. When you can painlessly use a dilator the size of your partner's penis, you may be ready for intercourse.

To order dilators online, see the Resources section.

HOW NOT TO TREAT PELVIC FLOOR PAIN

Do *not* . . .

- believe that your pain does not exist simply because it is not visible.

- settle for a physical therapist who is not knowledgeable in this field (see the Resources section for help finding one who is).

- be lax or casual about your home exercise program, which is crucial for your rehabilitation.

- neglect to make time for self-care.

POTENTIAL BREAKTHROUGHS: LOOKING TOWARD THE FUTURE

One very promising area of research concerns platelet-rich plasma (PRP) and other biologicals, which are taken from a person's own blood and then injected into her muscles, joints, or tendinous areas. This seems to be useful in combating tendon and muscle injury, almost like a tissue graft.

Healing muscle by applying different forms of energy—such as ultrasound and cold laser—is also something that is being researched, and we're gaining experience in it as well. Our orthopedic colleagues in the field of rehabilitative medicine are doing wonderful research on muscle injury and repair—all of which will lend itself to expanding the knowledge of and improving the treatment of pelvic floor muscle problems. Gait and movement abnormalities are also being studied, which will help us too. We expect that this type of sexual pain will be extremely well treated in the future.

Meanwhile, both Blair and Lucy have done very well with their treatments and are beginning to feel good about sex again. "I finally had my first orgasm with intercourse after more than two years," Blair reports. She admits that "the sex is still not where I want it to be," but she remains hopeful that she'll get back to the deeply satisfying sex she had before. And she has strong coping mechanisms. "What really helps me is paying attention to when I am feeling good, so when I go through more painful periods, I can look back and say to myself, 'I don't always feel this bad.'"

Lucy gleefully informed us that she can use a tampon again, and she's preparing to resume her sexual relationship with her boyfriend. She has begun to revise her sense of herself and to realize that the qualities that make her a sensual woman go beyond her genital equipment. "I realize now that when I first met Dave, he probably didn't go, 'Oh, what a great vagina that woman has,'" she says with a grin. We are glad she understood that her partner had fallen in love with her charm, her sense of humor, her perseverance, her exuberance, and her intelligence—not her vulva. "Not having sex has definitely affected Dave," Lucy says. "But I realize that it hasn't fundamentally changed his feelings for me. That's good to know."

11

PAIN RESULTING FROM ORTHOPEDIC CAUSES

I remember feeling so horrible and scared, thinking I didn't know how much longer I could tolerate this unending itching and burning in my vulva. I consider myself to be an extremely strong and capable woman, and I have faced many challenges in my life, including watching my mother die at a young age. . . . But I thought, of all things, this was going to be the medical problem that would finally do me in. There were days that I could barely take care of my children. I was always a very active mom who loved playing games and sports with my kids. I did what I had to do like making lunch and making sure my kids did their homework. But much of the time, I lay around with ice packs in my crotch, praying to God to end this horrible suffering. I also felt incredibly guilty that I couldn't be the kind of mother I had been before. I prided myself on being an exceptional mother, and at that point, I felt like nothing more than a dishrag. Both the pain and guilt were killing me.

—BETH, FREELANCE WRITER, LATE FORTIES

ORTHOPEDIC PAIN: AN OVERVIEW

Your back might hurt, or perhaps your knee, hip, or leg. Or perhaps you have an abdominal ache that seems to include both your muscles and your genitals. Maybe you're fine except for when you assume particular positions, or perhaps you hurt all the time. Possibly you're aware that an accident or injury was the original cause of your pain, or maybe you've just started to put two and two together. Or perhaps the orthopedic insult was more subtle, or the result of long-term wear and tear, so that you can't pin down when or how the problem started.

However your orthopedic problem began, you are now suffering during sex, and perhaps at other times as well. You may even be surprised to learn that your problem has an orthopedic source. This is one of those times when knowledge definitely is power.

The term "orthopedics" refers to the system of bones, joints, and associated tissues that enable the bones to move. Once again, we need to look closely at the amazing pelvis to understand how orthopedic dysfunction might translate into sexual pain.

The pelvis is enclosed by a mantle of bones and joints, and we will show how any may be the source of sexual pain. Illustrations 11-1 and 11-2 will help you visualize the structures we will be describing in this chapter. The lumbar spine (at about waist level), the sacrum, the coccyx (tailbone), and the top of the hip bones form the back of the pelvis. The front of the pelvis is held together by the pubic bone, while the side of the pelvis is formed by pubic bones and the hip joint.

If any of these structures is out of alignment, vulvar or pelvic pain can be the result. Tears or injuries in the joints and bones also can inflame the surrounding tissues, often irritating the nerves leading to the vagina and vulva. As with other types of sexual pain, we get a cascade of effects: bone or joint injury or misalignment affects muscles and tissues, which in turn affects nerves. Problems that began outside the vulva ultimately end up causing sexual pain.

Illustration 11-1.

PELVIC ORTHOPEDIC STRUCTURES

① Lumbar spine
② Sacroiliac joint
③ Sacrum
④ Pudendal nerve
⑤ Sacrospinous ligament
⑥ Acetabulum
⑦ Head of the femur bone
⑧ Psoas muscle
⑨ Coccyx
⑩ Pubic bone
⑪ Pubic symphysis
⑫ Obturator internus muscle
⑬ Iliopsoas tendon

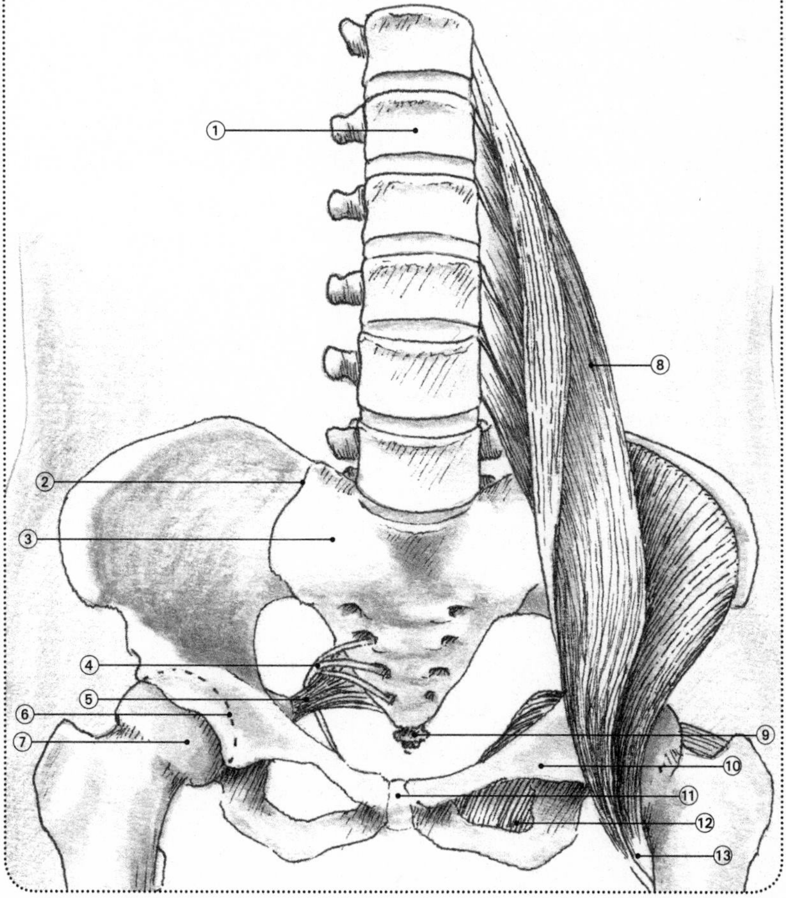

Illustration 11-2.

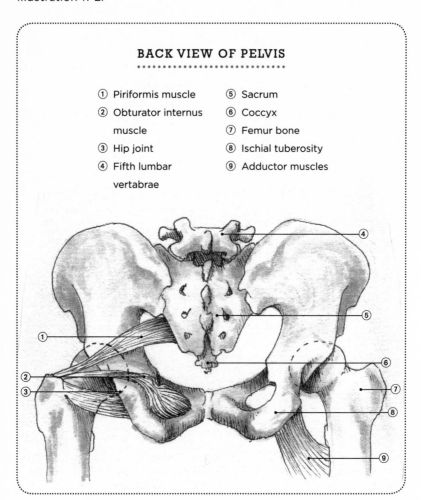

BACK VIEW OF PELVIS

① Piriformis muscle
② Obturator internus muscle
③ Hip joint
④ Fifth lumbar vertabrae
⑤ Sacrum
⑥ Coccyx
⑦ Femur bone
⑧ Ischial tuberosity
⑨ Adductor muscles

SYMPTOMS OF ORTHOPEDIC PROBLEMS

If your sexual pain has an orthopedic cause, you are likely to have one or more of the following symptoms:

- clitoral or deep rectal pain and/or itching when sitting;

- a deep, sharp pain in the vagina during penetration, usually on one side;

- stiffness in the legs, back, and/or hips in sexual positions;

- uncomfortable clicking of the hip, back, or groin when moving;

- in certain positions, sharp, radiating pain to the outer thigh, sometimes down to the knee, foot, groin, or buttock; and/or

- the inability to sleep on a particular side due to pain.

Women who have back disorders causing sexual pain may experience one or more of the following symptoms:

- numbness in the vagina during penetration;

- bladder and bowel problems;

- burning pain that worsens in certain sexual positions;

- sciatic pain, which radiates down the back of a leg; and/or

- tingling sensations in the groin or lower abdomen (if nerve roots from higher up are involved).

➤

Symptoms of a hip problem include the following:

- insidious pain in the front part of the hip and in the lower quadrant of your abdomen, as well as groin pain; pain may radiate to the thigh or knee;

- decreased range of hip motion as a result of pain and/or impingement;

- dull or sharp, constant or intermittent pain in the hip, often with clicking, pinching, and/or locking;

- pain that gets worse with activity, with prolonged sitting, when rising from a seated position, or when climbing stairs; and/or

- very weak gluteal muscles (buttocks).

Another potential indicator of hip problems is a history of one or more of the following activities:

- long-distance biking or "spinning";

- a job that requires prolonged sitting (because the hip remains in flexion too long);

- sports that use the hip in extreme flexion and abduction with quick stops and starts, including soccer, weight lifting, lacrosse, tennis, and field hockey;

- ballet or other types of professional or intensive dancing; and/or

- gymnastics, competitive cheerleading, or other activities that involve lots of jumping and falling.

HOW ORTHOPEDIC PAIN AFFECTS YOU

Orthopedic problems can severely affect your life by causing you pain every time you move. As a result, you avoid certain types of movement—or perhaps even all movement. In order to avoid pain, you start to "splint" your muscles—tensing them to keep the bones and joints from moving. This in turn causes them to weaken and perhaps even to atrophy. The weakness tends to generalize to the rest of the body, and you become progressively more uncomfortable in even the most ordinary of activities: sitting, walking, exercising. Even when you're not in pain, your deconditioning affects your sense of sexual well-being.

WHAT'S GOING ON: THE BIOLOGY

Have you ever seen a skeleton or a picture of a skeleton as it dangles from a string? Think of how all the bones fit neatly together, and how loose and flexible the joints are. When all the components of our skeleton are working well, we can stretch, flex, and move smoothly. We feel strong, balanced, and at ease in our frames. We can exercise as we please and assume sexual positions without fear.

But when any portion of our skeleton is injured, the effects radiate outward to affect our other bones and joints—as well as attached muscles and connective tissue, and then our nerves. Ultimately, we're looking at both the musculoskeletal system and the nervous system as pathways for sexual pain.

Let's zero in on the specific areas of the musculoskeletal system and the types of injuries that are most likely to create sexual pain.

The Back

The nerves that supply the vulva and vagina with motor and sensory signals leave the spine from the lumbar and sacral areas as nerve roots. As a result, any problem in this part of the spine can cause sexual pain—including injuries, scoliosis, osteoarthritis, bulging disks, cysts (fluid-filled sacs arising from the small vertebral joints), or tumors. And because these nerves supply the muscles and allow muscle function, injuries here can also cause muscle changes in the pelvis, which in turn can lead to pain.

Here are some key sources of back distress:

- Injuries to your lower back or disks can cause pressure on the nerve roots as they emerge from your spine and extend into your pelvis.

- Back surgery, such as spinal fusion, can cause sexual pain, due to scarring or other damage to the lumbar or sacral nerve roots that supply your pelvis through your ilioinguinal, genitofemoral, or pudendal nerves.

- If the coccyx (tailbone) is injured, you may feel extreme pain during penetration.

The Hips

Some women have a hip disorder that coexists with sexual pain—and that may also be the pain's actual underlying cause. The hip disorder may affect your movement, which in turn creates an imbalance in your muscles, thereby irritating your nerves and creating pelvic pain. That's why identifying a hip disorder can be extremely helpful, since restoring normal hip function corrects what may have triggered your cascade of pain.

Since the hip and pelvis share many of the same muscles, and since these muscles affect pelvic and vulvar nerves, it makes sense that sexual pain can result from hip disorders. While we don't expect you to remember the names of all the important muscles and nerves that are involved in orthopedic sexual pain, we're listing them here so you'll recognize them when you see them again. Muscles: piriformis, obturator internus, and iliopsoas. Nerves: pudendal, obturator, sciatic, ilioinguinal, iliohypogastric, genitofemoral, and sympathetic plexus. You can find many of these structures in illustrations 11-1 and 11-2, and 5-1.

If you've injured your hip, you've made subtle but important changes in your gait and movement to compensate for discomfort, hip instability, and mechanical impairment (as in hip impingement, where bone keeps colliding with bone). As we have seen, this creates problems in your muscles—which may tighten, shorten, stretch, or weaken to keep your core and pelvis stable. The central nervous system subconsciously "recruits" these muscles to do this job, even though it may be inappropriate for them to behave this way. The fascia and other connective tissues are also tightened, or shortened, adding to the imbalance and discomfort. And these structures in turn pinch, press, stretch, or otherwise irritate your pelvic nerves, which send pain signals to the brain.

Here are some specific ways that hip injuries might cause sexual pain.

LABRUM TEARS

The hip labrum is a horseshoe-shaped ring of dense connective tissue that attaches to the bony rim of the hip socket to deepen, reinforce, and stabilize the socket, and to seal and protect the joint. Tears in this tissue (called "labrum tears") cause Femoroacetabular Impingement (see below) and also force the pelvic floor muscles to compensate by tensing and shortening, putting pressure on the pudendal nerve and thus causing sexual pain.

FEMOROACETABULAR IMPINGEMENT (FAI)

This is a common condition with two possible causes. In one, the ball (the head of the femur) rubs against or collides with the hip socket (the "acetabulum"); both can be seen in illustration 11-1. When the ball and socket rub against each other, they create a bump (a "callus") that limits the hip's range of motion, especially with regard to your leg's ability to flex and rotate inward. Alternately, an outgrowth or bump on the acetabular rim might limit leg flexion and rotating outward.

Either way, we're usually looking at a vicious circle, in which these bumps create even more friction and therefore may get bigger, causing ever-greater instability and inflammation in the hip joint—and ultimately, a permanent loss of cartilage. If your cartilage is rubbed away, you're at risk for osteoarthritis. Meanwhile, the bumps or calluses throw your muscles out of balance, make movement more difficult, and frequently lead to nerve irritation and pain.

EXTRA-ARTICULAR HIP DISORDERS

The structures surrounding the hip can also cause pain. Extra-articular ("outside the joint") hip disorders include:

- bursitis in the hip and groin (see "Iliopsoas Conjoined Tendon Pain and Bursitis," later in this chapter);

- osteitis pubis (see "Pubic-Bone Conditions," on the next page);

- adductor strain (the adductors are the muscles that connect your legs to your pelvis); and

- psoas syndrome (a strain in the large psoas muscle that connects your lower body to your hip).

These hip conditions are seen more often in women than men. Why? Part of the reason is that women have a shallower hip socket than men. Therefore, trauma to the area has a greater effect—and since the number of women athletes is on the rise, so is this kind of condition. But there are some other common reasons too, including the following:

- hip hyperflexion and abduction (widely separating the legs out and away from the midline) during labor or vaginal surgery;

- hip hypermobility (due in part to hormones, women are more flexible than men); and

- prenatal and postnatal developmental hip disorders (these anatomical abnormalities known as "hip dysplasia" are far more common in women).

Other Orthopedic Causes

Back and hip disorders are the most common orthopedic causes of sexual pain. But a number of other, often severe conditions may also give rise to this pain. Unfortunately, most doctors are not aware of how common these conditions are among women, and how often they may lead to sexual pain.

COCCYDYNIA: PAIN IN THE TAILBONE

This type of pain is due either to a congenital abnormality or (more often) to an acute or chronic injury that causes the tailbone to deviate—right, left, forward, or back—rather than extending straight down. The displacement causes pressure on branches of the pudendal nerve and also pulls on the pelvic floor muscles, causing muscle imbalance—which pulls even more on the coccyx (tailbone), causing more pain. When you have coccydynia, deep penetration can cause excruciating pain and can also make your condition much worse.

SACROILIAC JOINT PROBLEMS

The sacroiliac joints hold your back and pelvic bones together. When they're unstable—as they are in many women, due to laxity in the ligaments holding the joint together—you can suffer from pelvic floor pain. Often these joints are themselves affected by movement disorders arising from hip labrum tears and femoroacetabular impingement (covered previously in this chapter).

Remember, the pelvis is tightly interconnected and operates as one working unit. Tightness and discomfort in the pelvic floor may be due to the pelvic muscles' compensating for instability in the sacroiliac joints. So if a sacroiliac joint is distressed, you may feel pain anytime your pelvis moves— and particularly during the regular pelvic movement involved in sex.

PUBIC-BONE CONDITIONS

The pubic bone is vulnerable to low-grade injury in sports and other activities, and that leads to inflammation—which may spread to the pelvis, the bladder, and even the clitoris, causing sexual pain. In addition, the adductor muscles of the legs originate at the pubic bone, and if they and their tendons are injured (they may tear and swell), pubic bone inflammation may follow. Pain from this inflammatory condition may also relay to the groin, clitoris, and urethra during sexual activity.

The front of the pelvic bones are held together in the midline by a joint called the pubic symphysis, which opens markedly with pregnancy and childbirth. Sometimes it opens too much and becomes weak and unstable, causing significant postpartum pain in response to movement—pain that might continue for months or even years if inflammation continues. This is called osteitis pubis.

ILIOPSOAS CONJOINED TENDON PAIN AND BURSITIS

The long psoas muscle is a major core and hip stabilizer and flexor that runs behind the pelvic organs and combines with the iliacus muscle in the pelvis to form the iliopsoas conjoined tendon, as seen in illustration 11-1. These muscles and their tendon connect the front of the bones of the spine to the hip bones. Injuries, hip disorders, and back problems can cause this structure to become inflamed, tight, or shortened—making it unable to do its work easily.

As with other pelvic conditions, an inflamed iliopsoas conjoined tendon can affect related nerves, such as the genitofemoral, which supplies part of the vulva's sensation. When disordered, this nerve transmits pain signals to the brain during sex. In addition, psoas-muscle pain can be confused with endometriosis pain, since it has a similar location in the pelvis.

Other vulnerable areas around the iliopsoas conjoined tendon are bursas—fluid-filled sacs that work to counteract tension and friction at joints and tendons. If they become inflamed, however, bursas around the iliopsoas conjoined tendon or at the outer hip can create severe pain in the groin and vulva—this is called bursitis.

ISCHIAL-TUBEROSITY PROBLEMS

The ischial tuberosities—the "sit bones"—are the bottommost bones of the pelvis. We put a lot of pressure on them with long hours of sitting (which our bodies are not designed to do), and they're vulnerable to chronic injury from falls and other traumas—including those caused by long-distance biking and other vigorous activities.

Hip disorders can also involve the ligaments inserting into the sit bones. Since the pudendal nerve runs right behind the bones and ligaments, inflammation here can create significant pudendal-nerve irritation, and thus sexual pain.

OSTEOARTHRITIS

Osteoarthritis is a common inflammation of joints. It affects twenty million Americans—more than half of them women. Pain and stiffness from osteoarthritis may limit movement in parts of your body that are involved in sexual activity, such as your hips, back, neck, and hands. It may be the most frequent cause of sexual pain, especially as we get older.

COEXISTENT MUSCULOSKELETAL DISORDERS

Some of the orthopedic disorders in this chapter often coexist with one or more of the following musculoskeletal conditions (if this is true for you, keep in mind that *both* conditions need to be addressed for a full recovery):

- Connective Tissue Disorders, which are undergoing more research and new understanding, are genetic conditions that may lead to hypermobility of all the various connective tissues in the body. The effect in the pelvic floor, hips, and back may cause injuries, FAI, painful muscle spasms, and even nerve pain, as we discuss in Chapter 9. One patient, while pursuing a career in genetic counseling, was able to diagnose herself with one type, called Ehlers-Danlos Syndrome, Hypermobility Type (Type III). Now that we know the reason underlying her pain, she can move forward to getting better.

>

> - hernias in the groin;

- chronic tendon inflammation/scarring (known as either "tendinosis" or "tendinopathy") occurring anywhere in the pelvic floor, hips, or low back; and

- foot problems and leg-length discrepancy, affecting gait and thus pelvic muscle balance.

COMMON MISDIAGNOSES FOR ORTHOPEDIC PROBLEMS

MISDIAGNOSIS	HOW TO RULE IT OUT
Pelvic inflammatory disease	Cultures, blood counts, imaging studies, laparoscopy
Endometriosis	Pelvic exam, imaging studies, laparoscopy
Ovarian cysts/ fibroid tumors	Pelvic exam, ultrasound
Groin hernias	Exam, imaging studies
Renal colic	Urine analysis, imaging studies
Psychological illness	MD awareness/education

DIAGNOSIS: THE TESTS YOU NEED

Chronic sexual pain is one of the most commonly misdiagnosed and mistreated conditions in all of medicine. We've seen dozens of patients whose doctors didn't perform the correct diagnostic tests to properly identify their disorders—or, in some cases, didn't perform any tests at all but instead relied on a quick look. This section is to help you ensure that your physician is ordering the right tests to create a good diagnosis and treatment plan. If he or she is not ordering these tests, you probably want to consider finding another doctor.

Diagnosing orthopedic injuries and disorders is often relatively straightforward, but what is not so clear is the link between these problems and sexual pain. Fortunately, a much better understanding of the links between hip and back and pelvic floor is emerging, and more and more doctors are beginning to see that fixing the "unhappy" hip or back does often reduce sexual pain, or even make it go away. But unfortunately, curing orthopedic pain is not a quick fix, because it takes time to get your core strong and in balance again.

For these often somewhat mysterious or confusing orthopedic conditions, your physician should be working with a team of experts, since no single MD can know or do it all.

The Basics

Your doctor's first step should be to take a detailed history from you. This is always an important part of diagnosing sexual pain, but it is particularly so with orthopedic causes, since a certain amount of detective work is needed to identify the initial injury. In fact, taking a good history may be more important than any test.

Often, orthopedic pain does not seem to stem from any trauma. However, sports or other injuries can suggest orthopedic problems, as can lifestyle—such as a pattern of prolonged sitting, dancing, or other types of vigorous or repetitive movements. Infancy and early-childhood hip problems are also risk factors for adult hip problems. Hip discomfort at any time, present or past, might also be clues to orthopedic problems.

A detailed physical exam will also be very helpful. Your doctor should observe your gait, as a high percentage of women with orthopedic problems walk with a mild intermittent limp. Have your doctor evaluate your hips and back in standing position as he or she looks for tenderness, asymmetry, deformity, and scoliosis (curvature of the spine).

Diagnosing Hip Injuries

We have at our disposal a number of physical-exam maneuvers to see if the hips are "unhappy." The easiest of these include:

- the FABER (Flexion, ABduction, External Rotation) test, used to identify decreased rotation or pain when the hip rotates outward;

- the flexion–internal rotation–adduction impingement test, used to identify decreased rotation or pain when the hip rotates inward; and

- palpation of the greater trochanter (the outer part of the hip), which looks for tenderness and bursa problems.

Your doctor should also conduct a careful pelvic exam, with special attention to the hip-related anatomy. During the vaginal and rectal exams, your doctor should assess, by feel, the obturator internus muscle, a primary hip rotator that is depicted in illustrations 11-1 and 11-2, to show how it connects the hip to the pelvic floor. We have found that this muscle bears a lot of strain when the hip is weak, unstable, or impinged and off-balance. It attaches to the other pelvic floor muscles and may greatly affect them. When we examine the obturator internus, hip and potential pelvic floor problems are often indicated by the following symptoms:

- tenderness, tension, tight bands;

- an increase in resting tone;

- asymmetry between right and left sides; or

- hypertrophy (overgrowth) or atrophy (shrinking).

Your physician should also test the pudendal nerve at the sacrospinous ligament complex at the ischial spine (see this landmark in illustration 11-1). When touched gently with an examining finger, a distressed nerve will respond with pain, often radiating to or referred to another part of the pelvis—or even to the hip or buttocks.

If your history and your response to this type of pelvic exam suggest hip problems, your doctor may proceed to imaging studies: x-rays, ultrasounds, MRIs, or CT scans (though we try to avoid the latter because of radiation). Your doctor may choose a study based on what's available in your community. However, MRIs are the most helpful, since the soft tissues surrounding the bones and joints are easily seen on the new high-resolution scans. They may show signs of labrum tears, impingement, inflammation, or swelling in the tissues around the hip joint. The newer scans can also image the obturator internus muscles and reveal the course of the pelvic floor nerves. Abnormalities here help prove the link between your hip and sexual pain.

Diagnosing Other Problems

A history and a physical exam are key first steps for diagnosing other orthopedic problems, as is imaging. However, we need to keep in mind that "when we look, we find." As people get older, many "normal" changes occur in bones and joints that could look like serious problems on x-rays or MRIs, especially if the radiologist interpreting them has no knowledge of the patient's age, history, and physical exam. For instance, some studies show that up to 30 percent of people in general without back or hip pain will show some degree of abnormality in an MRI of these areas, and these changes will be noted in their reports. This percentage will go up the older we get as our tissues go through normal "wear and tear." And we may walk around with these changes, feeling no ill effect at all. That's why you need the help of good, experienced orthopedic specialists to evaluate your test results, and interpret them in light of your individual symptoms and pain, before a treatment plan can be recommended. In addition, each of us has a different anatomy and gait, and we all use our bodies differently in our work and personal lives. These differences also put us at risk for different types of joint and spine problems, as do our genetics and childhood histories. Keeping this big picture in mind is often critical to identifying the problems causing your sexual pain.

Diagnostic Injections

Specialists will often recommend a diagnostic intra-articular hip injection or injections into inflamed tendons or muscles. Using x-ray or ultrasound guidance to pinpoint the correct location in your pelvis, a specialist will administer an injection combining numbing and anti-inflammatory medications.

In particular, this approach can offer remarkable relief for hip labrum tears and FAI, as well as for associated vulvar and vaginal pain. Although the pain relief may not occur for one or two weeks, any reduction in pain suggests that your hip is indeed involved in your sexual pain.

The contrary, however, is not true. If you undergo a diagnostic injection and receive no relief from pain, you may still have an orthopedic disorder, but your pain may be the result of changes in the surrounding muscles, fascia, and nerves.

Specialists can use similar injections to test for lower-back problems too. These may include:

- "facet joint injections" into areas where one vertebra connects to the next;

- injections into the muscles that surround the spine and that may be pulling on the disks or squeezing down on nerves;

- epidural injections; and

- spinal nerve blocks.

For coccydynia, injections into and around the coccyx may be helpful diagnostic tools. Diagnostic injections are also available for such structures as ligaments and tendons attaching to pelvic bones and joints—including the adductors, iliopsoas conjoined tendon, gluteal muscles, sacroiliac joint and surrounding ligaments, sacrotuberous ligament, ischial tuberosity, and pubic bone.

TREATMENTS: WHAT YOU CAN EXPECT

Sometimes an orthopedic problem requires a rapid or extreme response, as in the case of one of our patients, who was found to have a lumbar spine fracture that had gone undiagnosed for years. This injury was now causing such severe nerve compression that she was at risk for permanent nerve damage and numbness. Luckily, the expeditious back surgery she underwent led to a complete recovery.

Such "rapid-response" cases, fortunately, are the exception. You are far more likely to have several treatment options, and you should begin with the least invasive, progressing to more complicated treatments only if you have to.

Conservative management—such as muscle rest and lifestyle changes—is usually the first option, but by the time you're experiencing sexual pain and reading this book, we can assume you've moved well past this stage. Nevertheless, you should be trying to avoid abnormal movements in order to reduce inflammation and muscle imbalance. For example, if you have a hip problem, you need to avoid prolonged sitting, moving your legs to extreme positions, and stressful repetitive motions. For back problems, avoid lifting, unbalanced bending, and poor posture. For coccyx and sit-bone pain, avoid sitting, and use a padded seat cushion if you must. Acupuncture and yoga may also be helpful for these problems.

Anti-inflammatory medications such as ibuprofen and naproxen will help your joints heal, along with the surrounding muscles, ligaments, tendons, and cartilage. Topical anti-inflammatory or lidocaine skin patches can also be helpful. In some cases, oral muscle relaxants can keep muscles from overworking and going into painful spasm. Pain medications might also help you to walk more normally, removing the strain on the problem area. (However, be careful of opioids, as this type of pain medication may create more problems than benefits for you.)

SETTING REALISTIC GOALS

A lot of times, for patients, it is all or nothing: They want to be back to where they were years ago, and they forget how bad they were when they first started physical therapy.

But when you set specific goals for patients and review the goals periodically, you find that they have met many of them. It's like crossing something off a long to-do list. Their hope starts to come back when they find that they can sit in pants for work—when before they couldn't even think about putting on pants—and when they are able to become intimate with their partner. Setting goals and giving time frames and revisiting past goals—reminding women of where they were compared to where they are now—gives them great hope. They realize how much better they are now. They will have an ongoing sense of hope that they will continue to get better, and that the pain will get manageable. Taking those baby steps is important.

Everything has to be done slowly and precisely. Patients who want to become intimate with their partner must remember: You can't run a marathon without walking first. You must start slowly and then begin to run. You need time, and you need to realize everyone has the same goal for you: to decrease your pain. But you must start slowly, and as you make progress, you'll realize how you will get much better.

—STACEY FUTTERMAN, PT, MPT, BCB-PMD

Physical Therapy

Whatever other types of pain relief you employ, your mainstay of treatment for most orthopedic problems is almost certainly physical therapy. In our experience, most women improve enough from this approach that they don't need invasive therapy. That's because physical therapy can attend to all the connections within the pelvis that tie a problem in one location to pain in another. In our experience, some three-quarters of our patients find physical therapy effective.

However, physical therapy does not offer a quick fix. You'll need to invest a minimum of three to six months. To make this commitment, you need to buy in wholeheartedly to the concept that getting your pelvis stronger, aligned, balanced, relaxed, and moving correctly is your key to success in healing your sexual pain. You'll need to work even more than the average patient in physical therapy, since your pain has probably debilitated you both physically and mentally.

We understand that when you're tired and feeling weak, just the thought of doing your home exercises seems too much to bear. Try to remember that, besides reducing your sexual pain, physical therapy can help you turn a corner in your general health—that the way to live longer and better is to exercise and stay strong.

Make sure your therapist understands how to rehabilitate both your orthopedic problem and your pelvic floor. You might even need to see two physical therapists who can work together to cover both areas. Your treatment goals will include:

- normalizing your pelvic floor muscles;

- mobilizing the fascia, other connective tissue, and even skin of the hips and lower back;

- strengthening the hip and core muscles, including the gluteal muscles, which often become extremely weak;

- relaxing the obturator internus and piriformis muscles, taking pressure off pelvic nerves; and

- fixing gait and movement abnormalities—all the way down to your feet.

Minimally Invasive Treatments

Moving up the scale to more-invasive treatments, the injections discussed in the diagnosis section can also be helpful as treatments. For example, some of our patients have gotten six months or more of relief from intra-articular hip injections.

Other treatment options are cold laser, ultrasound, dry needling, and trigger-point injections to muscles in pain or spasm due to imbalance. Many physiatrists and physical therapists use this approach in conjunction with physical therapy.

Surgical Options

If none of these approaches succeed, you might consider surgical options: for example, arthroscopic hip repair of labrum tears and femoroacetabular impingement, or back procedures like microdiscectomy. If these surgeries help you walk without pain and lessen strain from your daily activities, your muscle balance will improve, and your sexual pain will decrease.

After any orthopedic surgery, it's crucial that you continue physical therapy for at least six months. Now that your hip fits better into its socket, or your lumbar disk is not pressing on a nerve, you have the chance to retrain and rebalance your pelvic floor muscles to work normally. But this retraining takes time. Some women notice that they are not better for a year, because improvement is gradual and they were so weak before. Others note great improvement after only two or three months. Your recovery depends on the severity of your condition and the degree of pelvic imbalance that was causing your pain.

Surgical complications are rare, but they do exist. They include infection, deep vein thrombosis, anesthesia side effects, and scarring of connective tissue. Your outcome is best if your surgeon is very experienced in the particular type of surgery you need, and if you approach your recovery with the energy and commitment required to heal well.

HOW *NOT* TO TREAT ORTHOPEDIC PROBLEMS

Do *not* . . .

- ignore your sexual pain—if your conditions worsen, your treatment options may be more limited.

- ignore the possibility that your back or hip pain is connected to your sexual pain.

- overexercise or exercise without guidance, since you might worsen an imbalance.

- go to a chiropractor who is unfamiliar with the relationship between the pelvis and the back.

- use untested herbal treatments made in China for such conditions as joint pain, as these may have toxic contaminants.

POTENTIAL BREAKTHROUGHS: LOOKING TOWARD THE FUTURE

The future is very, very hopeful for healing orthopedic problems causing sexual pain, as research is advancing rapidly to devise less-invasive means to treat these problems. Physical therapy techniques are improving; the individuality of our bodies is being recognized; and newer substances to optimize healing are being studied.

For example, platelet-rich plasma (PRP) is being used to locally regenerate injured tissue, as are stem cells—and these techniques will soon come into wider use. Surgical procedures for helping orthopedic problems are also advancing rapidly—becoming less invasive and requiring less post-op downtime. And the role of preventing further injury in women with orthopedic conditions will become better recognized, so that sexual pain will not be an outcome of these problems.

Beth, whose story you'll read about in the "complicated patient" section of Chapter 16, has had an unusually difficult healing journey, with numerous complications after her initial orthopedic problem (a tear in her hip labrum). Most other patients with orthopedic pain face far easier and more straightforward recoveries than Beth. But even she has not given up hope.

"I know that I have gone through hell and back, and I will never forget the emotional and physical pain that I had to endure. I don't plan on becoming embittered by my experiences but instead plan on using what I have learned to be there for other women who are going through similar experiences," she says. "And one message I want to convey to other women is that they should not go through this alone. Reach out to other women, or get professional help. This is too much to bear alone."

12

....

PELVIC ORGAN
PAIN AND
ENDOMETRIOSIS

I saw two doctors who put me on two different antibiotics, even though I tested negative for urinary tract infections. After being on the antibiotics, not only was my pain untouched, I developed a yeast infection. I saw three other doctors—none of whom could help me, and all of whom made the problem worse by what they prescribed. I was so sick of seeing all these specialists who couldn't help me. It seemed like every time a doctor gave me another medication or treatment recommendation, I got worse or developed another problem. I was not only depressed but I was also becoming really scared—what if there was no one out there who could help me?

Now it's been six years, and I still have flare-ups. My pain level varies, but it is much more pronounced when I urinate. Then I feel like I have a chopping pain in my vulva. There are days when I am going to the bathroom every ten minutes. There are days when I am unable to leave the house. And this puts a tremendous strain on my marriage, because my life is sometimes so restricted, and then my husband suffers.

—LISA, GUIDANCE COUNSELOR, AGE THIRTY-FIVE

Two weeks before my wedding, I was diagnosed with a horrible vaginal infection and was put in the hospital. I definitely think that stress makes things worse. I had this vaginal infection for seven months—bladder pain, vulvar itching, and stabbing pain. And my urinary frequency went through the roof. At that point, I had to go to the bathroom every fifteen minutes, and had to get up eight or nine times a night.

Can you imagine being newly married and having to deal with this? I was so depressed at this point and thought my vaginal infection would never go away. I felt completely helpless and felt that nothing would work to help me. I never seriously contemplated suicide, but the thought crossed my mind that the only break I was going to get from this pain would be when I was dead.

—KAREN, FASHION DESIGNER, LATE TWENTIES

PELVIC ORGAN PAIN: AN OVERVIEW

Your bladder hurts, and it burns when you urinate. Or your stomach hurts every time you're stressed, and you struggle with constipation, diarrhea, or both. Or you're bleeding—as though you had a perpetual period—far too much and far too often, with a nearly constant pain from menstrual cramps. Or your abdomen hurts—intermittently or all the time, but always in mysterious ways from causes you can't identify. Your muscles in your pelvis, back, and abdominal wall may ache at the same time. And all of these painful, frustrating conditions are accompanied by pain before, during, or after sex.

You are suffering from a disorder of one or more of your pelvic organs: painful bladder syndrome (PBS), irritable bowel syndrome (IBS), endometriosis, uterine fibroids and/or adenomyosis, or pelvic congestion syndrome (PCS). To better understand how the organs involved in these types of sexual pain live closely together in the pelvis, see illustration 12-1.

Illustration 12-1.

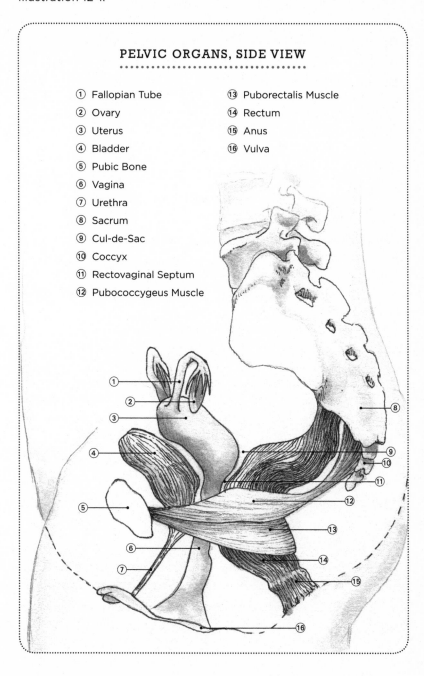

PELVIC ORGANS, SIDE VIEW

① Fallopian Tube
② Ovary
③ Uterus
④ Bladder
⑤ Pubic Bone
⑥ Vagina
⑦ Urethra
⑧ Sacrum
⑨ Cul-de-Sac
⑩ Coccyx
⑪ Rectovaginal Septum
⑫ Pubococcygeus Muscle

⑬ Puborectalis Muscle
⑭ Rectum
⑮ Anus
⑯ Vulva

Your physician may or may not have correctly diagnosed these stubborn, painful, and chronic conditions. But if you do have a diagnosis, in some cases, the doctor does not think your diagnosis is linked to your sexual pain—even though it is. In other cases, the doctor does think your diagnosis is linked to your sexual pain—even though it isn't. That said, you have lots of reason for optimism: All of the conditions in this chapter can be treated. But you may be facing a long road to full recovery.

SYMPTOMS OF PELVIC ORGAN PAIN

The following are symptoms of painful bladder syndrome:

- intense bladder pain during vaginal intercourse;

- urgency to urinate during and after intercourse;

- pain flares that result from sexual touching;

- urinary frequency that may last several days after sex;

- the constant feeling of needing to urinate, even after just emptying;

- a frequency of urination that disrupts sleep; and/or

- a knifelike pain during urination.

Irritable bowel syndrome has the following symptoms:

- frequent pelvic/abdominal bloating that makes intimacy uncomfortable;

- gas pockets that hurt;

- residual pelvic discomfort after intercourse;

➤

- pelvic floor pain with sex; and/or

- anal pain with sex, due to skin irritation or anal fissures.

The following are symptoms of endometriosis:

- stabbing pain with intercourse, felt deep in the pelvis;

- during your period, severe cramps or backache;

- bladder pressure that is worse premenses and with menses;

- cyclic bloating and worsening of symptoms; and/or

- pelvic tenderness (residual pain) after intercourse for hours or days.

The following are symptoms of fibroids or adenomyosis:

- a feeling of heaviness and fullness in the pelvis;

- sometimes irregular or very heavy menstrual bleeding; and/or

- deep pain with intercourse or penetration.

Symptoms of pelvic congestion syndrome are:

- pelvic heaviness on one or both sides, increasing as the day goes on;

- heaviness and discomfort that become worse with upright activities;

- deep discomfort with penetration, which may persist as residual pain for hours; and/or

- a worsening of the condition before and during menses.

COMMON MISDIAGNOSES
FOR PELVIC ORGAN PAIN

MISDIAGNOSIS	HOW TO RULE IT OUT
Recurrent bladder/ urethra infection	Specific bacterial cultures
Ovarian cysts	Pelvic exam, ultrasound
Pelvic inflammatory disease	Cultures, blood counts, imaging studies, laparoscopy
Groin or abdominal hernias	Exam, imaging studies
Lumbar spine disc disease	Physical exam, imaging studies, nerve studies
Overactive bladder syndrome	Symptoms persist after treatment; may coexist
Psychological illness	MD awareness/education

HOW PELVIC ORGAN PAIN AFFECTS YOU

Painful Bladder Syndrome

If you suffer from painful bladder syndrome, you may feel anything from mild discomfort, pressure, and tenderness, to intense pain. The pain may occur with, before, or after urination, or may be continuous.

One version of the pain is a constant feeling of needing to urinate, even after just emptying. Frequency of urination can also disrupt your sleep many times in a night, causing major sleep deprivation, which in turn saps you of the energy you need to handle your pain. All of these symptoms often become more pronounced during certain phases of a woman's menstrual cycle, especially premenstrually.

According to Karen—the patient quoted at the beginning of this chapter—the hardest thing is how the seemingly constant need to urinate and the periodic urgency of the need to urinate come to dominate your life. Painful bladder syndrome can result in a woman needing to urinate as often as sixty times throughout a single day and night. Ordinary activities at work and in the world become organized around the need for bathroom breaks and the importance of remaining close to a bathroom at all times. Conversations and phone calls are interrupted; errands become a challenge; and long drives and long walks in nature are out of the question. Many women feel embarrassed to excuse themselves for a bathroom break, especially multiple times, and many of our patients have reported extreme fatigue and fogginess from sleep disturbances.

Lisa (also quoted at the beginning of the chapter) told us she sometimes felt like she was going out of her mind because her symptoms so severely limited her daily activities. "I feel pressure from my bladder constantly," she says. "I have the feeling that I constantly have to go. Sometimes I can't even leave my house."

Painful bladder syndrome can affect your life in more subtle ways as well. "One big thing that is hard for me is my restrictive diet," says Karen. "I can never have alcohol, which I feel affects me socially. I was never a big drinker. But three or four years ago, I was very depressed about this restriction. When you go out with friends, you socially drink, and the fact that I couldn't held me back socially. It also made me very angry and spiteful that my husband and I would go out, and I would always be the designated driver. I always felt that everyone was having fun, and I wasn't," she says.

"Another aspect of my life that is very difficult for me is my two-hour commute to work. I've found that the seats on the train are not good for me and possibly were causing some nerve damage. If I sit for too long a time, my urethra goes into spasms and my vulva problems get worse. I use a special pillow at work, but it's not portable, so I can't take it on the train."

Karen now sits in the club car of the train, where the seats are more comfortable, and she has organized her social life in ways that don't include drinking. But she continues to be frustrated by how often she has to accommodate her medical condition.

Many women find it particularly upsetting to have to go to the bathroom so often, particularly when they have to interrupt making love to do so. For single women, especially, it can be a challenge, as many find the situation difficult to explain.

Irritable Bowel Syndrome

A key aspect of irritable bowel syndrome involves the close relationship of the brain and the gut. Normally, psychological stress affects our bowels—fear produces diarrhea, for example—but ideally, the relationship is regulated, so that mild stress, anger, or fear does not immediately affect the gut.

In IBS, that relationship is "dysregulated," so that even minor stress causes instant and perhaps intense pain. Moreover, we've recently begun to understand that the gut has its own "brain," producing many of the brain chemicals (including serotonin) that affect our mood, sleep patterns, and general well-being. Irritable bowel syndrome affects our intestines' ability to produce these natural antidepressants, with painful results.

This condition can have an astonishingly far-reaching impact on your daily life. Studies have shown that it is a significant cause of absenteeism and decreased work productivity. For example, one team of researchers found that 15 percent of IBS sufferers in the United States had changed their work schedule, while 25 percent worked fewer hours. Another study reported that IBS patients missed three times as many days from work as people without the condition.

Here are some other ways that IBS might affect your daily life:

- Your time-management skills and your ability to concentrate may be affected.

- Because of the demands of your intestines, you may need more time for your commute.

- You may be reluctant to go out for a meal or take a long trip.

- You may have a harder time taking or enjoying holidays, especially if they involve going to unfamiliar places and being away from a private bathroom.

- You may anticipate bloating pain, which affects your ability to enjoy eating, socializing, and destressing activities.

- You may become unduly anxious about the need to have a bowel movement before you leave the house or while you are gone, which might limit your social and/or professional activity.

Because the bowel is in the pelvis, any distress there is likely to translate into sexual distress as well. Here are some examples.

- Frequent pelvic or abdominal bloating can make touch, penetration, and other intimacy uncomfortable.

- Genital skin may be irritated from contact with diarrhea.

- Anal tears and fissures caused by constipation may produce sexual pain.

- Constipation may make intercourse painful because of the hard stool in the rectum, just behind the vagina.

- Residual pelvic floor muscle discomfort after intercourse is common among women with IBS, given that so much of the pelvis is irritated, inflamed, and tense.

PELVIC ORGAN PROLAPSE

A common problem for women is abnormal relaxation and weakness of the pelvic floor muscles, tendons, and fascia—often due to heavy lifting and/or obstetrical injuries stemming from the vaginal delivery of a large baby, with associated tearing of the tissues. As we get older, the pull of gravity, genetic predisposition, and muscle de-conditioning all contribute to the development of bulging sensations at the vaginal opening. This feeling is from a lower position of the uterus, bladder, or rectum in the pelvis and may come with low back ache and overactive bladder or loss of urine with a cough, sneeze, or during sex. Many urogynecologists focus their practice on the surgical repair of these annoying and occasionally medically risky problems.

We mention POP here because a moderate or severe degree of prolapse can certainly cause uncomfortable feelings of looseness, fullness, and even lack of sensation with penetration. Pelvic floor physical therapy can do wonders for these symptoms, and make surgical repair (if needed) more successful since your muscles will be stronger. However, POP is rarely the cause of significant chronic painful sex, so if you are diagnosed with POP and told that surgery for mild or moderate uterus or bladder prolapse will cure your painful sex, *please get a second opinion*. You very well may have one of the many other conditions we have covered in this book, which means that you could be left with the same pain—or even more pain—after surgery.

Endometriosis

Deep pain with intercourse is a characteristic feature of the painful sex that pelvic endometriosis may create. In all but the mildest cases, endometriosis implants grow in the cul-de-sac and rectovaginal septum of the pelvis (see it depicted in illustration 12-1), causing inflammation, loss of tissue elasticity, and extreme tenderness to touch here. This is the exact pelvic area that is touched by the deep thrusting of your partner's penis. Our endometriosis patients describe themselves "hitting the ceiling" from the stabbing pain they may experience during intercourse, often making it impossible to continue.

Fibroids and Adenomyosis

You may experience pelvic discomfort, a distended abdomen, or heavy bleeding—all of which can affect your sense of well-being. If the bleeding is heavy and frequent enough because of a fibroid in your uterine lining, your daily life (particularly at work) becomes compromised by efforts to avoid "accidents."

Generally, these conditions should not unduly affect your sex life. However, if either is severe enough, you may experience the following sexual effects:

- pressure during sex, due to a bulky uterine mass;

- avoidance of certain sexual positions in response to the pressure of a large fibroid; or

- feeling less free and spontaneous in your sex life due to tenderness, heavy bleeding, or bladder pressure.

If the fibroids or adenomas are especially large, you may notice fatigue, backache, discomfort due to the bulkiness of the enlarged uterus—or anemia if you are losing a lot of blood.

Pelvic Congestion Syndrome

The general sense of heaviness and the intensification of menstrual discomfort from PCS may dampen your interest in or ability to enjoy sex. In addition, you may experience deep pain with intercourse or penetration. The condition may also keep you from being able to stand for long periods of time, due to the pain you may feel as the pelvis "fills up" during the day.

WHAT'S GOING ON: THE BIOLOGY

There are several organs within the pelvis, including the bladder, bowel, uterus, fallopian tubes, and ovaries (see illustration 12-1). Each has its own disorders, with its own symptoms, diagnoses, and treatments.

To understand how your pelvic organs can cause so much pain, recall our discussion of the nervous system of the pelvis in Chapter 9. As we saw, the pelvis is special in that many of the autonomic nerves that control the pelvic organs travel with the nerves that carry sensation from muscles, skin, and connective tissue. These two types of nerves overlap and interconnect in the spinal cord, and without the brain knowing it, can mix their signals. An impulse that begins in an organ (for example when your bowel is bloated from gas) may get sent via the spinal cord to the pelvic floor muscles, causing them to brace and become tense, resulting in pain both sexual and otherwise. The brain then has trouble consciously relaxing these muscles to override this reflex. Often this muscle tension spreads as your core tries to adapt, causing more pain in the lower back or the psoas muscles, and resulting in connective tissue problems. In order to heal your pain, we need to tease it apart and approach it from both angles—your distressed pelvic organs and your pelvic muscles.

Meanwhile, *if you have any one of the following organ conditions, you are likely to have one or more of the others,* since they share nerve pathways and hormonal triggers (often tied to the menstrual cycle), and since there is so much cross-talk among them in the central nervous system. We suggest that you first read about your primary symptoms, diagnosis, and treatment, then go through the rest of the chapter to see if you have one of the other conditions as well.

Painful Bladder Syndrome

The bladder is an expandable muscular sac located in the lower abdomen, just behind the pubic bones and in front of the vagina. When your bladder is working properly, it's a wonderful organ: quietly storing urine until it's time to empty via the short canal called the urethra; self-cleaning as it empties, so that you avoid infectious bacteria; and doing nothing to interfere with sex.

When your bladder is not working properly, you may be frequently and unhappily aware of it, especially during sex. One key disorder that may cause you problems is known as painful bladder syndrome (PBS). (An older medical term—interstitial cystitis—is also still used.) This condition is commonly misdiagnosed as a repeated urinary tract infection (UTI) because the symptoms may be exactly the same. Unfortunately, the antibiotics used to treat UTIs aren't helpful in resolving painful bladder syndrome and might even make the condition worse.

Some two million U.S. women have PBS, along with four million women who suffer from a related condition known as overactive bladder. Both names describe a group of symptoms that include discomfort or pain in the area of the bladder and the surrounding pelvis, most often with frequent urination.

PBS seems to be triggered by an injury to the lining of the bladder—or, like vestibulodynia, it may be present from birth. Irritating chemicals in the urine move through the abnormal bladder lining into its underlying layers, causing inflammation and nerve irritation. In longstanding cases, fibrosis (a buildup of fibrous, scarlike connective tissue) and loss of elasticity in the bladder muscle make it even more painful to fill your bladder. Although the source of the original injury remains somewhat mysterious, frequent UTIs are involved. There is probably also a genetic or developmental component.

As discussed in Chapter 10, pelvic floor dysfunction may be both a cause and an effect of painful bladder syndrome. Some women with pelvic floor dysfunction find that the muscles surrounding the urethra and bladder base become too tight, pressing on and constricting these structures and their nerves. Pain and the need to frequently urinate are the result. Conversely, many women with PBS go on to develop imbalance and tension in the pelvic floor muscles. This may result from reflexively gripping these muscles as a response to the bladder pain, and from the complex nerve interconnections between organs and muscles in the pelvis and spinal cord. In fact, up to 80 percent of women with PBS suffer from pelvic floor dysfunction, and vice versa. Vulvar pain, irritable bowel syndrome, and endometriosis also frequently coexist with PBS.

Irritable Bowel Syndrome

Irritable bowel syndrome (IBS) is another very common condition believed to affect some 14 percent of the U.S. population—and twice as many women as men. Unfortunately, doctors are still far too slow in diagnosing this condition, and studies show that about one-fourth of all patients with this diagnosis had to visit a health professional at least five times in order to get it.

As with other conditions that cause sexual pain, a delay in diagnosis and therefore in treatment is very problematic, as pelvic floor muscles go progressively further out of balance, and nerves become "trained" to send pain signals up to the brain. The sooner this syndrome is caught and treated, the less extensive its negative effects will be (for instance, the less likely that muscles will also become involved). The greater the delay, the longer and more extensive the treatment process becomes.

Irritable bowel syndrome is a functional disorder of the intestinal tract in which motility (the tract's ability to move) is altered. Constipation and/or diarrhea are the result, as is a pain disorder that gives the visceral nervous system a heightened sensitivity. As a result, any movement of the tract—including that produced by gas and stool—is very painful, and bloating and distension often add to the pain. Significantly, IBS is usually relieved temporarily by defecation.

Although some of the symptoms of IBS may seem to resemble those of other bowel disorders, functional brain MRIs show that the brain reacts uniquely in this condition. Like PBS, it often has a centralized component to the pain, as the spine and brain "rewire" and inappropriately keep the pain cycle active.

In our experience, if you take a careful history, a significant percentage of IBS cases—perhaps as many as one-fourth—begin with a gastrointestinal infection that does not fully improve. IBS that includes constipation frequently creates pelvic floor disorders, due to the effect of retained hard stool on the pelvic floor muscles and also due to the frequent straining to defecate. Likewise, anal fissures are very common. Both the fissures and the tightening of the pelvic floor are painful—and both can then make the IBS worse. In addition, stress can cause relapses or flare-ups.

Irritable bowel syndrome commonly coexists with:

- painful bladder syndrome;

- fibromyalgia;

- endometriosis;

- chronic headaches (perhaps because of low serotonin levels); and/or

- vulvar pain syndromes.

Endometriosis

Endometriosis is a common condition. Over 5.5 million U.S. women have it, and 60 percent of women with endometriosis suffer from what can be the most extreme form of sexual pain.

Endometriosis occurs when cells that normally line the uterine cavity appear elsewhere in the pelvis—most commonly on the fallopian tubes, ovaries, and peritoneum (the lining of the pelvic cavity). We aren't completely sure what causes this condition, but the latest research gives good evidence that it is present at birth in 11 percent of all women, and that it arises from stem cells residing in the peritoneum. Estrogen, which increases at puberty, stimulates growths from these cells, in tissues that were not designed to support them. The resulting inflammation, nerve proliferation, autoimmune reactions, and fibrosis in the endometriotic implants create severe cyclic pain in the pelvis, and produce pain with penetration.

Endometriosis often occurs between the uterus and the bladder, on the uterosacral ligaments (which link the uterus to the spine), in the peritoneum deep behind the uterus (the cul-de-sac), and in the rectovaginal septum (the tissue between the vagina and rectum). (See illustration 12-1.) The inflammation and scarring of these tissues cause various pelvic structures to adhere to each other, so that they can barely move.

Recently, we've come to appreciate that endometriosis may create inflammation as well as abnormal fascia and other connective tissue in the pelvic floor. This leads to other changes in this area as well, such as the alteration of blood and lymph flow through the scarred layers, and sometimes the development of enlarged blood and lymphatic vessels. As a result, local nerves are restricted and irritated, providing another potential source of sexual pain.

Surgeons are often the primary doctors treating this condition. But since surgeons, by nature of their specialty, often have a limited treatment focus, many women have told us that they are left to fend for themselves when it comes to treating their associated medical symptoms—especially their sexual pain and hormonal-medication side effects.

Fibroids and Adenomyosis

We don't want to give the wrong impression about these conditions. Although they are frequently blamed for sexual pain, fibroids and adenomyosis are rarely responsible for it. These conditions, along with ovarian cysts, are common; they can often be felt during an exam; and they are easily visible with imaging. As a result, physicians have often latched onto them as explanations for sexual pain. The treatment for these conditions is mostly surgical, so unfortunately, many women—including many of our patients— have undergone unnecessary surgeries in the hopes that fixing these conditions would help with sexual pain. Then, after surgery or other medical treatments fail to relieve the sexual distress, women are often told that their pain must be all in their heads—literally adding insult to injury.

These conditions are very rarely the main or sole cause of severe or long-lasting sexual pain. We urge you to be very skeptical about any doctor who tries to convince you that they are.

Fibroid tumors (scientifically known as leiomyomata uteri) are benign tumors of the uterus that develop from the smooth muscle cells. They can occur singly or in multiples—up to dozens in some women. They appear in all sizes and in all locations in the uterus. They're very common: Up to 45 percent of all U.S. women in their forties have fibroids when evaluated by ultrasound; for African American women in their forties, that figure rises to 65 percent.

Adenomyosis is a related and common condition in which glands that usually just line the uterine cavity grow in the wall of the uterus, either in one area or diffusely throughout it. Like fibroids, it is often blamed for sexual pain, though it rarely causes it. However, when fibroids or adenomyomas are large, lowlying in the pelvis, or going through a process called degeneration (a dying off of the inner cells), they may be responsible for some deep sexual pain. As a result of the close connection between the nerves serving the organs and those serving muscles and other tissue, these structures may refer pain, causing distress in other areas of the genitals and in the pelvic floor.

Pelvic Congestion Syndrome

Pelvic congestion syndrome (PCS) occurs when damaged vein valves cause the pelvis or pelvic floor to become full of enlarged veins, like the varicose veins in our legs that many of us get as we age. These enlarged veins put pressure on organs, nerves, and the surrounding connective tissue.

DIAGNOSIS: THE TESTS YOU NEED

Chronic sexual pain is one of the most commonly misdiagnosed and mistreated conditions in all of medicine. We've seen dozens of patients whose doctors didn't perform the correct diagnostic tests to properly identify their disorders—or, in some cases, didn't perform any tests at all but instead relied on a quick look. This section is to help you ensure that your physician is ordering the right tests to create a good diagnosis and treatment plan. If he or she is not ordering these tests, you probably want to consider finding another doctor.

Painful Bladder Syndrome

A correct diagnosis of painful bladder syndrome should start with a process of elimination to rule out all other possible causes—such as urinary tract infections and other types of bladder or urethral disorders. Urine cultures to check for bacterial growth, urine analysis, and urine cytology (a microscopic examination of the bladder cells obtained from urine) to be sure there is no infection or cancer are key. An evaluation of the urethra (the narrow canal that carries urine from the bladder out of the body) by exam, and possibly by using a small visualizing telescope, is important if it is the site of pain, to rule out cysts and infections.

Bladder instillations via a urinary catheter are diagnostically helpful. In the past, potassium was placed in the bladder to see if pain was provoked—if it was, that would confirm PBS. More recently, and less painfully, we are using anesthetic agents. If pain is relieved, the diagnosis of PBS is highly suspected.

Nerve tests, such as small-fiber studies for neuropathic pain, may also help in planning treatment and ruling out other pain disorders. These tests are discussed in Chapter 9 under "Special Nerve Function Tests."

Sometimes, more-invasive procedures are needed to look within the bladder, such as cystoscopy—a telescopic view of the inside of the bladder, performed with or without anesthesia. Unfortunately, this procedure may trigger flares of pain, so tests must be chosen carefully.

We can't stress too strongly how important it is to move quickly to diagnose PBS. Young women with pain remaining after treatment for UTIs need to be recognized and treated without delay, as studies are showing that this is the best way to prevent full-fledged PBS. The longer the pain continues, the more aggressively it will need to be treated.

Irritable Bowel Syndrome

The first step in diagnosing irritable bowel syndrome is to rule out other bowel conditions. We make sure that the problem isn't parasites by testing stool. We rule out cancer or inflammation by testing for hidden blood. We look for digestive conditions such as gluten sensitivity and lactose intolerance, which frequently coexist with IBS in any case. We may also use blood tests to rule out leaky gut syndrome, a condition in which the intestine "leaks" undigested food into the gastrointestinal system, causing a kind of autoimmune response as the system becomes "allergic" to common foods.

We're also looking for potential vitamin or mineral deficiencies, as well as structural conditions, such as a long colon—though these are rare. Ultimately, because there isn't a chemical test we can administer to identify IBS, we rely on a patient's description of symptoms and their effect on her quality of life.

The generally accepted diagnostic criterion for IBS as of this writing is recurrent abdominal pain or discomfort for at least three days per month over the last three months, associated with two or more of the following symptoms:

- pain or discomfort that improves with defecation;

- an association between the onset of the pain/discomfort and a change in stool frequency; and

- an association between the onset of the pain/discomfort and a change in the appearance of the stool.

Endometriosis

Key to diagnosing endometriosis is a good history, especially of cyclic pain symptoms. You'll also need a physical exam to determine the classic signs of this condition, which are:

- low or no mobility of pelvic organs when your physician tries to move them;

- nodules (tender bumps) detected during a deep pelvic and rectal exam, on your uterosacral ligaments and in your rectovaginal septum; and

- ovarian swelling called endometriomas (ovarian cysts made up of endometriosis).

Your physician may order imaging studies, such as a transvaginal ultrasound or MRIs—but often these do not reveal the tiny implants of endometriosis. A laparoscopy (surgical telescopic view of the inner pelvis) is the gold standard in both diagnosis and treatment.

Fibroids and Adenomyosis

Once again, a good history is crucial for your physician to be able to track your cyclic heavy bleeding and pain patterns. You will also need a physical exam so your doctor can identify an enlarged or tender and bumpy uterus. Imaging studies can then help zero in on a diagnosis. Transvaginal and pelvic ultrasounds are particularly important, as are MRIs, in difficult cases. As with any other pelvic growth, it is important for your doctor to rule out uterine or ovarian cancer with these tests.

Pelvic Congestion Syndrome

Your physician's first move should be to do a clinical exam, looking for tenderness in the area of your ovaries. To diagnose pelvic congestion, he or she will need a very high "index of suspicion" and should first rule out other pelvic organ and pelvic floor conditions.

The diagnosis can be further honed in on with imaging studies. Ultrasound is best but must be taken in a relatively upright position to allow your veins to fill. An MRI with contrast may also be helpful, but again, your position is important, because if you are lying down, the condition won't be as evident.

TREATMENTS: WHAT YOU CAN EXPECT

For all the pelvic organ conditions we discuss in this chapter, there are excellent treatments now available that will help your resulting painful sex. Each condition has its own individual treatment, but remember that you may be also suffering from pelvic floor pain, so be sure to read the treatments in Chapter 10.

Painful Bladder Syndrome

Our first line of treatment for painful bladder syndrome is dietary and life-style changes, to eliminate the stress and toxins that overtax the bladder, and to introduce nutrients that support its healing. Miraculously, in some cases, our patients' symptoms remit without any dietary/lifestyle changes or treatments at all. In most cases, though, a low-acid diet can go a long way toward eliminating symptoms, along with avoidance of caffeine (which is a diuretic), cigarettes, alcohol, cranberries (which are perhaps good for UTIs but not for PBS), and artificial sweeteners. Certain foods, including Bartlett pears and blueberries, help coat the bladder lining. We also recommend improving your sleep hygiene—since deep, restful sleep is such an important component of the healing process. A regular regimen of gentle stretching exercises helps too.

Medically speaking, we must acknowledge that there are no silver bullets for this syndrome. However, there are treatments that can calm the pain enough to allow you to have pain-free sexual activity and to go about your life.

Our first effort is always to locate all the sources of pain—known as "pain generators"—and to attempt to relieve each one separately. Potential pain generators include pelvic floor muscles, nerves, the urethra, and the bladder itself.

As in other sexual-pain conditions, it is important to treat muscles with physical therapy, since, as we have seen, the nerves for muscles and organs are so intimately bound up with one another. We use soft-tissue mobilization around the urethra and the base of the bladder to improve the connective tissue. We also retrain the bladder, using schedules to promote regular urination and to accustom the bladder to being filled. We have you chart your intake of liquids, to see if we can help you regulate bladder input to a comfortable, steady flow.

Local medications can also greatly help to relieve pain. Topical and vaginal hormonal creams and suppositories help strengthen the urethral mucosa, which may have become irritated, inflamed, and painful. Topical anesthetics applied to the urethra before you empty your bladder can prevent pain. Diazepam (Valium) used as a vaginal suppository, as well as other muscle relaxants, can help ease the reflexive gripping of the pelvic floor muscles in response to pain. As we saw in the diagnosis section, bladder instillations via a urinary catheter can allow us to apply several medications to calm the injured bladder lining. Pentosan polysulfate (Elmiron)—used either orally or via instillation—helps to coat the bladder lining and prevent further irritation.

Oral medications can also bring relief from pain. Antihistamines like hydroxyzine work on the inflammatory chemicals made by the injured bladder lining. Sleep aids for nocturia (frequent nighttime urination) can help you get the healing rest you need. Nonsteroidal anti-inflammatories (aspirin, ibuprofen) can ease the pain. Also helpful are bladder medications that in the past were mostly used for overactive bladder or for men; these include anticholinergics (oxybutynin, for example), antispasmodics such as hyoscyamine and flavoxate (Urispas), and alpha adrenergic blockers like tamsulosin (Flomax).

In addition, treating the nerves with oral medications is often a key component of relieving PBS. Nerve-sedating medications such as serotonin–norepinephrine reuptake inhibitors (SNRIs), tricyclics like amitriptyline (Elavil), and antiepileptics can calm the nerves that are sending amplified pain signals to the brain. Opioid-like drugs like tramadol are also in our toolbox, but we have found that the benefits of regular narcotic painkillers are far outweighed by the problems they create.

We can also administer pain medications by injection around nerves supplying the bladder, such as the pudendal nerve and sympathetic nerve ganglions in the pelvis. Sacral nerve stimulation—also known as sacral neuromodulation—is now a well-studied treatment in which the amplified bladder-pain signals are "scrambled" as they enter the spine, decreasing their "volume" and impact by the time they register in the brain. This technique has helped a significant number of PBS sufferers.

Other types of injections may also be useful. Botulinum toxin A (Botox) injections can help restore balance to overly tense pelvic floor muscles around the urethra and base of the bladder. Botox injections into the bladder wall through cystoscopy may also calm an overactive bladder.

Consider a trial of the birth-control pill if your symptoms seem to worsen cyclically, as minimizing the ups and downs of your hormonal levels might rid you of some hormonal triggers to the syndrome.

If less-invasive treatments don't succeed, then you may need to move on to surgery. Cystoscopy with hydrodistention (expanding the bladder capacity forcefully with water) may help severe cases. In a very tiny minority of the most severely disabling cases, more extreme procedures exist to reroute urine. But the vast majority of PBS sufferers do respond to the treatments listed above, so don't lose hope and jump to these types of invasive treatments.

THE IMPORTANCE OF DISCIPLINE AND PATIENCE

There is much research now showing that manual therapy is key to the patient's recovery. It is vital to stick to the program with regard to muscle reeducation—once or twice a week, plus a home exercise program every day—to help bladder issues heal. Some home exercises for bladder dysfunction include certain stretches of the pelvic floor, hips, abdominal muscles and back muscles. Relaxation and breathing exercises help the muscles too.

We are very realistic with patients, telling them they should not expect to be going to the bathroom only every two hours after the first physical therapy treatment. It is a slow process. If someone is going to the bathroom every fifteen minutes, our goal for the next week may be to try to make it every twenty minutes.

>

> > *We must make realistic short- and long-term goals. It is important for the patient and doctor to be on the same page here.*
>
> > —AMY STEIN, PT, MPT, BCB-PMD

Irritable Bowel Syndrome

All treatments of irritable bowel syndrome must be multimodal to address the bowel, nervous system, and pelvic floor components. Exercise is crucial for good bowel function and for your overall sense of health. You also need to regulate your fluids, making sure to drink six to eight glasses a day of water, juice, or herbal tea. But do not overdo the fluids, as this can put a strain on your gastrointestinal system, and avoid carbonated beverages, since they increase bloating. Likewise, eat a moderate-fiber diet—but avoid too great an intake of fiber, as that can also worsen bloating. Since dietary fat can inhibit intestinal motion, a low-fat diet is best.

You can regulate the firmness of your stool with stool softeners. You've got lots of safe and natural options, so engage in a little trial and error to find the one that's best for you.

Probiotics and some medications can help improve bowel motility, while other medications may treat your pain component. Among others, lubiprostone (Amitiza) may be of benefit if your IBS is constipation-dominant. Very recently, studies are showing that about one-fourth of all IBS patients benefit from courses of rifaximin (Xifaxan)—an antibiotic that is nonabsorbable, meaning that it remains in the intestinal tract and does not enter the bloodstream. This quality makes it safe and worth a trial.

Because IBS can disrupt serotonin production, the class of antidepressants known as SSRIs—selective serotonin reuptake inhibitors—may be able to help regulate your body's supply of this crucial bowel and brain chemical. Due to this close brain–gut connection, in which every emotion or stressful thought may be felt in the gut, hypnosis and cognitive–behavioral therapy have very significant benefits for people with IBS. (See the Resources section at the back of this book.) Likewise, any form of stress reduction, including yoga and meditation, can be extremely therapeutic.

If you're suffering from anal fissures, pelvic floor physical therapy can be very helpful in restoring normal function and balance to the muscles around your anus and rectum, so as to promote the easier passage of stool. Topical medications, injections, and Botox may also be used to treat the perianal muscles, helping to heal fissures.

Overall, your IBS is manageable, and the sexual pain it causes can be helped.

Endometriosis

An entire book could be written on treating endometriosis. Make sure to see the Resources section at the back of the book to find ways to obtain more information.

First, surgical excision of all endometrial tissue is necessary. Your best chance for a total cure will be attained with an expert surgeon who has the skills to completely remove all of the abnormal endometrial tissue and to release adhesions and remove scar tissue—rather than a surgeon who treats only with laser, cautery, or other less-complete techniques. Your deep sexual pain will only be helped if the difficult excision of the cause—the deep cul-de-sac and rectovaginal endometriosis—is performed. Many less-knowledgeable or undertrained gynecologic surgeons do not appreciate the necessity of doing this, leaving you with the same pain after your surgery. We have seen patients who have undergone ten or more surgeries before finally improving with the appropriate excision. This skill unfortunately is not obtained in medical school or residency training, but must be learned through special fellowships or collaboration with an already-expert surgeon.

The good news is that techniques are improving, and we look forward to the education and training of more surgeons to facilitate your access to the best surgery. The use of robotic surgery may allow the learning curve to move faster and less expensively for more surgeons. And doctor–patient collaborative support groups are spreading the word about this disabling condition (see the Resources section at the back of the book).

Some 60 percent of women are greatly helped by surgery, but that means that about 40 percent need further treatment. Like women with other types of sexual pain, endometriosis sufferers are often demoralized, even hopeless, by the time they receive a correct diagnosis and effective treatment. Meanwhile, medications that moderate the fluctuations of estrogen may keep residual endometriosis from growing back, but they have significant side effects. Fortunately, the negative effects of these hormonal therapies are also treatable.

We urge you to begin pelvic floor physical therapy for your tense muscles, and for soft-tissue mobilization, which will treat remaining adhesions and tissue scarring and restrictions, and which will increase the blood supply to the organs and tissue. You can relieve pain with nonsteroidal anti-inflammatory drugs (NSAIDs) such as aspirin or ibuprofen. Some opioid agonists, such as tramadol (Ultram), may be effective for severe pain (but use them with caution). Complementary and integrative medicine will offer you a holistic approach that includes diet, exercise, good sleep, and stress reduction.

Fibroids and Adenomyosis

Pain medications—including nonsteroidal anti-inflammatory drugs and opioid agonists—are helpful. Hormonal medications that can decrease your estrogen levels, reduce the size of uterine fibroids or adenomyomas, and stop menses should also be considered. Physical therapy with soft-tissue mobilization helps to treat adhesions and nerve restrictions and to increase blood supply to the organs and tissue.

If you are close to menopause, be aware that your fibroids will quiet down dramatically when your menses stops.

Complementary and alternative treatments have actually been quite helpful for these conditions. Acupuncture in particular can be an effective way to treat the symptoms of both fibroids and adenomyosis.

Finally, if your sexual pain and quality-of-life problems continue, you might consider one of several surgical techniques to remove your fibroids and adenomyomas.

HOW *NOT* TO TREAT PELVIC ORGAN PAIN AND ENDOMETRIOSIS

Do *not* . . .

- delay endometriosis treatment.

- consider your cyclic symptoms too "routine" to treat.

- fail to obtain second opinions for surgical approaches.

- cheat yourself by not considering physical therapy.

- avoid treatment for fear of hormonal medications (if carefully planned and followed up on, they are safe).

Pelvic Congestion Syndrome

Your first line of treatment is a trial of hormonal medication. One choice is a course of medroxyprogesterone acetate, a synthetic progesterone, for four to six months. Oral contraceptive pills or leuprolide (Depo-Lupron) and similar medications may also help to shrink the veins hormonally. Nonsteroidal anti-inflammatory analgesics may be used for pain. As always, physical therapy is helpful—in this case, with a core-strengthening focus, to improve muscle tone, which will better support the veins and pelvic structures.

Among other techniques, laparoscopy to cauterize the veins is a possibility if medications don't work as desired. Working with an interventional radiologist, your physician might consider embolization of the veins to block them off: A thin catheter is passed into a groin vein and then on to the varicosities using x-ray guidance; then a blocking medication is delivered, clogging off the veins permanently.

POTENTIAL BREAKTHROUGHS: LOOKING TOWARD THE FUTURE

We've looked at a diverse group of conditions in this chapter, but they all have one thing in common: Advances in a number of medical fields are progressing rapidly, offering a lot of hope to women who do not obtain adequate relief from current treatments.

In hormone research, for example, there are many new studies on manipulating hormones safely without side effects, to treat and prevent these conditions. Progesterone antagonists (blockers) are one example. New surgical techniques using robotics are being developed to bring relief with minimally invasive procedures. Advances in anti-inflammatory approaches will be useful for all the conditions in this chapter. And sacral neuromodulation has been found to be very helpful for visceral pain—that is, organ pain that involves the autonomic nervous system and the complexities of cross-talk among nerves.

Our patients are also hopeful. Karen may not be able to drink alcohol when she goes out, but she still has an active social life and enjoys the company of friends when she goes out to dinner. Lisa has regained some of the romance and intimacy she and her husband shared before her condition began, and she is hopeful that things will continue to improve. Both women believe that though their lives have been altered, they still have a good quality of life and look forward to improvements in their conditions.

13

HORMONAL
AND OTHER CAUSES
OF PAINFUL SEX

My problems began about fifteen years ago, when I started meno-
pause. Several physical changes happened simultaneously. I started
to develop inflammatory arthritis, which made my joints very sore.
And then, gradually, I started to develop pain with intercourse.
When we had sex, it felt like someone had cut my vestibule.

I had always enjoyed sex, and before I met my husband, I had
a lot of boyfriends. I thought sex was the best thing since sliced
bread. But when I reached menopause, and I tried having sex
with my husband, it felt like I would tear more each time. It hurt
tremendously.

—STEPHANIE, RETIRED BANKING EXECUTIVE, AGE SIXTY

HORMONAL, SYSTEMIC, AND SURGERY-BASED
PAIN: AN OVERVIEW

You feel burning and tearing whenever anyone touches your vaginal opening, and sometimes you have irregular menstrual bleeding. Or perhaps you
feel burning and stinging when your urine touches your delicate tissues.
You're struggling with hormonal difficulties, postpartum vaginal spasms, or

menopausal sweating and sleep deprivation. Or perhaps you're coping with diabetes, an autoimmune condition, or the aftereffects of surgery or cancer treatment.

Hormonal, systemic, and surgical causes for sexual pain are among the most common and frustrating to deal with—largely because these conditions are difficult to begin with, and because most physicians don't make the connection between them and sexual pain.

We'd like to reassure you on two counts. First, the problem is not in your head: There are demonstrable medical connections between hormonal, systemic, and surgical conditions and sexual pain. Second, you absolutely *can* be helped, although you may need a lot of patience to heal both the underlying condition and the sexual pain. It may take a while to rebalance your hormones, stabilize your autoimmune condition, or restore your health after surgery. It may also take time to find the treatments that will fit both the underlying problem and the sexual pain. It can be done, though, so please don't give up—and read on to find out more.

SYMPTOMS OF HORMONAL AND SYSTEMIC CONDITIONS

You may feel these symptoms after pregnancy, when estrogen levels drop abruptly and remain low until breastfeeding is over. You may also feel them after menopause, a hysterectomy or other surgical procedure, in response to cancer treatments, or due to systemwide or autoimmune conditions:

- burning and tearing at the vaginal opening with touch, sometimes accompanied by small amounts of bleeding;

- discomfort in response to touch and/or tight clothing;

➤

- change in discharge to a thin, yellow type that may feel very irritating;

- stinging of urethra and surrounding skin during urination, along with more frequent urination;

- weakness in the pelvic floor muscles;

- a painfully tight feeling in the muscles during or after intercourse; and/or

- uncomfortable spasms in the vaginal muscles with sexual touch.

During pregnancy, you may feel the following symptoms:

- puffy and swollen labia that feel uncomfortable with sex (your labia actually enlarge physically);

- an overly wet feeling (at the vaginal opening) with stinging and itching with touch; and

- an aching in pelvic floor muscles with intercourse.

Occasionally, sexual pain is the presenting symptom of fibromyalgia. "Myalgia" means "muscle pain"—which, in this condition, may appear in the pelvic floor muscles and fascia. If you also have the following systemic symptoms alert your doctor to examine you for the signs of fibromyalgia (such as bodywide tender points):

- fatigue;

- sleep disturbances;

- stiffness; and/or

- cognitive problems.

HOW HORMONAL, SYSTEMIC, AND SURGICAL CAUSES OF SEXUAL PAIN AFFECT YOU

If you're struggling with hormonal changes, systemic illness, or postoperative recovery, you may not realize that your sexual pain is part of these larger conditions. You may also feel drained and discouraged by any of these other conditions, leaving you with little energy to cope with the sexual pain—even though it is adding to your demoralization and perhaps depression. Again, we urge you not to give up—treatments are available—and to strengthen yourself with good nutrition, restful sleep, and psychological support.

WHAT'S GOING ON: THE BIOLOGY

Our endocrine system, which produces our hormones, and our immune system, which is designed to protect us from harmful organisms, control, integrate, and coordinate our complex reproductive processes from a distance through our bloodstreams. These systems may develop problems, and when not functioning well, can imbalance or deplete our pelvic organs, leading to sexual pain.

Hormonal Causes

Our female hormones are critically involved in the health of our vulva, vagina, pelvic floor muscles, fascia, and pelvic organs. So when your hormones are out of balance, your sexual and pelvic health will be as well.

Hormones are chemicals that are made by our bodies in one organ or tissue. They are released into the bloodstream and travel to other organs, causing physiological responses there. The key female hormone, of course, is estrogen, which is integral to our sexual health and well-being—as well as to our menstrual and reproductive cycles and to our passage into menopause. Estrogen is also central to our overall health: Every tissue of our entire body (even connective tissue) contains estrogen receptors, which bind this hormone when it arrives via our bloodstream. Estrogen is likewise crucial to the function of our brain, our most important sex organ.

As you can see, disruption to and changes in female hormone levels can affect our entire bodies and our brains—and can therefore lead to changes that cause sexual pain, such as the following:

- thinning of the surface tissues of the vestibule and vagina;

- shrinkage of the labia;

- drying, due to reduced vaginal and sexual secretions, which allows little tears to occur with intercourse;

- thinning of the urethral and anal openings;

- sensitivity of the vulvar skin, causing discomfort with touch;

- shrinking and shortening of the pelvic floor muscles, because lower estrogen levels decrease blood supply and nutrients to them;

- compromised pelvic floor fascia, which loses elasticity due to insufficient estrogen;

- bladder and bowel dysfunction, since their support structures require estrogen; and

- decreased sexual desire and arousal, and difficulty reaching orgasm, since estrogen and testosterone are crucial for those responses.

The most common and extreme natural hormonal alterations in women's lives occur with pregnancy, childbirth, and the menopause transition, so if you have begun feeling sexual pain after any of these changes, you are very likely responding to the hormonal shift you are undergoing.

Other hormonal changes can be induced by medical interventions, such as hormonal treatments (including birth-control pills) and other treatments, especially surgery that removes the ovaries, our major estrogen producer.

To be sure, most women don't experience significant sexual changes, let alone pain, with hormonal shifts. But some do seem to be exquisitely sensitive to these effects, especially those that come with lowered estrogen levels. Studies estimate that some 50 to 75 percent of menopausal women undergo distress from vaginal changes—though about half of these distressed women say they learn to live with them. Unfortunately, only about 10 to 20 percent say that their physician ever asked them about this problem.

What this means is that if you're one of the women suffering from hormonal changes, you'll have to be very proactive about getting a proper diagnosis and treatment.

POSTPARTUM HORMONAL CHANGES

Having a baby is a wonderful phase of your life, but it can also be a scary time—for both you and your partner. If you're breastfeeding, you are living in a special hormonal milieu that for most women creates a low libido—even more than you might expect from just being tired after middle-of-the-night baby care. Your partner may also feel less sexual because of fatigue, anxiety over the life change, or the stress of a changing identity—or because seeing a partner as a parent can change the sexual dynamic. Combined with these factors, any sexual pain after childbirth can put a real stress on your relationship.

If a decreased interest in sex, or actual discomfort from sex, continues beyond the first two months, we urge you to seek help from your doctor. Your sexual problems are worth treating, because even though most women feel better when they get back to regular menstrual cycles after weaning, some women develop problems with their pelvic floor, which may worsen if they continue to have intercourse despite sexual pain.

For some postpartum women, the situation is even more complicated. Their tissue is delicate—not only because of hormonal changes, but also because they have sustained lacerations, muscle tearing, nerve injury, or trauma to the pubic bone or coccyx. There is treatment for these problems, as we explain in Chapters 10 and 11, and you need to make time for yourself to get the help you need. Remember, even your baby will be happier if you are happy: Many recent studies have shown that a mother's stress can affect the emotional health of her baby.

Of course, if you've had sexual pain before pregnancy, the possibility of having painful sex after giving birth may be very frightening for you. But we have good news: Many sexual-pain sufferers improve during and after a pregnancy—perhaps due to the increased blood flow, beneficial hormonal effects, and the relaxation and lengthening of muscles and fascia. So try sex again if you can, but have your doctor check out any pain—or worsening pain—as soon as possible if it occurs.

HORMONAL CHANGES RESULTING FROM CANCER TREATMENTS

Although cancer treatments save lives, they are often an added cause of sexual pain. Many women with breast, uterine, or ovarian cancer have undergone surgically induced or chemotherapy-induced menopause. They are the ones who undergo the most severe symptoms and sexual pain, because the hormone change is so sudden, and the entire body and brain—not just the pelvis and vulva—are shocked by the change.

Breast cancer treatments in particular can induce or exacerbate vulvo-vaginal pain. There are 2.6 million women alive today who have had or still have breast cancer, according to the U.S. Centers for Disease Control, and current treatment for the condition requires most to remain on aromatase inhibitors (such as Femara, Arimidex, or Aromasin) for at least five years after their breast cancer diagnosis. These medications prevent virtually any estrogen from being made in the body. As a result, the vulva and vagina atrophy—a significant source of painful sex, and for a huge number of women in our country. And sadly most of these women are not informed by their medical oncologists that this predictable pain should be expected, and can be safely treated.

Chemotherapy for any type of cancer can also lead to sexual pain, as it decreases ovarian function and adrenal function and greatly decreases both estrogen and testosterone. As we saw in previous chapters, female genitals need testosterone as well as estrogen. Since our adrenals manufacture up to 50 percent of our testosterone and related hormones, adrenal dysfunction can cause a significant decrease in testosterone, either temporarily or permanently.

ONCOSEXOLOGY

If you've had cancer of any type, it has almost certainly affected your sexual functioning at some point—especially if your cancer relates to your breasts, ovaries, or uterus, but also if it doesn't. Even when doctors are aware of these connections, these topics are often very difficult for them to discuss. Studies have shown that even gynecologists bring up postoperative sexual functioning only 40 percent of the time when their patients have had surgery for gynecological cancers. The topics of sex, cancer, death—all remain virtually off-limits, uncomfortable for doctors and patients alike.

Fortunately, a new medical discipline has been born: oncosexology, concerned with improving the sexual lives of people surviving or living with cancer. For women in particular, this is a crucial concern, as some seven million U.S. women are currently cancer survivors, and 25 percent of all women living today are expected to develop cancer in their lifetimes. About half of these will have a distressing change in their sexual function and intimacy, largely due to sexual pain.

The field of oncosexology is giving new attention to the long, productive decades now possible for millions of people after cancer diagnosis and modern successful treatment. This field is promoting awareness, research, and training of professionals to provide better care to those who need and deserve it, especially women suffering from painful sex.

Systemic Causes

Just as hormones travel in our bodies from one organ to another, so do other biochemicals, particularly those involved in inflammation. A number of systemic conditions that create inflammation can also trigger sexual pain because of their biochemical effects on all your organs, including your genital organs.

The biochemicals involved are produced by cascading autoimmune responses in the tissues and include various types of antibodies and cytokines—some of which even cause the abnormal function of nerve endings. They create pain in normal body tissue; decrease blood supply to the organs; produce scarring and abnormal fascia and other connective tissue; and irritate and sensitize nerves. These inflammatory, autoimmune conditions include:

- celiac disease (gluten-sensitive enteropathy);

- chronic fatigue syndrome;

- dermatomyositis;

- fibromyalgia;

- Hashimoto's and Graves' thyroid disease (which also cause hormone imbalances);

- multiple sclerosis;

- myasthenia gravis;

- Sjögren's syndrome;

- rheumatoid arthritis;

- systemic lupus erythematosus; and

- type 1 diabetes.

These conditions have some symptoms in common—including fatigue and pain—but each tends to affect the genitals in different ways.

For instance, diabetes tends to restrict blood supply to the genital nerves, leading to neuropathy and nerve pain. Dermatomyositis, fibromyalgia, and myasthenia affect muscle function, leading to pelvic floor pain. Skin and underlying fascia inflammation are common in lupus and Sjögren's, leading to surface vulvar and vaginal pain.

Because of these kinds of differences, you need to work with a physician who is either aware of how your condition can produce sexual pain or who

is willing to self-educate. Once you understand which types of sexual pain
may be created by your condition, you can also refer back to the appropriate
chapters in this book.

Diagnosis of these conditions is often based on blood tests that show
inflammation and abnormal autoimmune antibodies. Treatments are varied,
but we recommend having a good MD partner in rheumatology to help you
keep your underlying condition under control, which will be crucial to helping alleviate your sexual pain.

Surgical Causes

Many surgeries produce physical changes that cause sexual pain. In addition,
some women feel disfigured by surgery, which affects their sexual function
even more.

Pelvic surgeries are obviously the most likely candidates for producing
sexual pain, including surgeries for the following:

- vulvar cancer;

- prolapse of vagina, uterus, bladder, or rectum (Pelvic Organ
  Prolapse);

- direct nerve injury at time of C-section, hysterectomy, or laparoscopy, or due to neuromas forming in scars from these
  procedures; and

- sling procedures for urinary incontinence, especially those done
  with the use of a "mesh," which can cause painful tissue erosion
  in over 3 percent of cases.

Also, sometimes a hysterectomy will have the effect of shortening the
vaginal canal, which may lead to sexual pain from scarring and from difficulty accommodating a partner.

If you have had surgery for cancer, you might be given postoperative radiation therapy, which can knock out ovarian function and cause

menopause and its changes (see "Hormonal Changes Resulting from Cancer Treatments," earlier in this chapter). Radiation also causes scarring, as well as nerve and blood-vessel changes—which can in turn affect the bladder and intestines, possibly causing painful bladder syndrome and irritable bowel syndrome (see Chapter 12). You may experience these changes up to three years after treatment, often making them difficult to trace back to their initial cause.

Hormonal changes may also occur from surgery, causing the same types of sexual pain as a very rapid menopause. For example, if a woman has both ovaries removed—because of cancer, endometriosis, or infection—we call it "surgical menopause." If you haven't already gone through this process naturally, you will experience the most severe and sudden type of menopause: rapid-onset vulvar–vaginal atrophy and systemic illness, complete with hot flashes, sleep disorders, muscle and joint stiffness, and possibly depression and suicidal thoughts.

FEMALE GENITAL CUTTING

Studies estimate that some 228,000 women now living in the United States have undergone some form of female genital cutting. This has been considered a rite of passage for centuries for many girls in parts of Africa, and varies from cutting away a small portion of the skin at the clitoris to removing most of the labia and clitoris. Most of these women don't have sexual pain, but if you do, excellent minor surgical procedures exist to help relieve your discomfort. Many of these procedures can be tailored to your preferences, including the way that you prefer to look. See the Resources section if you want to find out more.

COMMON MISDIAGNOSES
FOR HORMONAL AND SYSTEMIC PROBLEMS

POTENTIAL CONDITION	HOW TO RULE IT OUT
Recurrent genital herpes	Magnified exam of the vestibule, herpes cultures, blood test for herpes antibodies
Recurrent yeast infection	Wet smear, specific fungal culture, or DNA test
Recurrent bladder/ urethra infection	Specific bacterial cultures
Painful bladder syndrome	Cystoscopy
Vulvar skin disorders (i.e., lichen sclerosis)	Magnified exam, biopsy
Psychological illness	MD awareness/education

DIAGNOSIS: THE TESTS YOU NEED

Chronic sexual pain is one of the most commonly misdiagnosed and mis-treated conditions in all of medicine. We've seen dozens of patients whose doctors didn't perform the correct diagnostic tests to properly identify their disorders—or, in some cases, didn't perform any tests at all but instead relied on a quick look. This section is to help you ensure that your physician is ordering the right tests to create a good diagnosis and treatment plan. If he or she is not ordering these tests, you probably want to consider finding another doctor.

For hormonal conditions, your physician should find it easy to see the drying and thinning of your vulvar skin, as well as the redness and thinning of the vestibule and of the vaginal and urethral mucosa. He or she may observe smaller labia and clitoral structures, a contracted vaginal opening with decreased elasticity, and a tenderness to touch in all these structures. Also visible may be tiny tears in the posterior fourchette (the V-shaped structure at the back of the vestibule) and, sometimes, chronic deep fissures from repeated tearing from intercourse. Overall, the tissues are likely to appear dry, and perhaps there will also be thin, yellowish vaginal secretions.

Essential to diagnosis is a wet smear and a pH test of vaginal secretions, which will reveal a lack of lactobacilli (the "good" bacteria) and a lack of mature surface-type vaginal cells, along with a preponderance of the basal or deeper cells and a high pH. This imbalance shows thinning and an actual loss of the stronger top layer of the vaginal lining, such as a burn would cause. There may also be white blood cells, which shows a degree of inflammation. Other helpful exams include hormonal blood tests, to confirm a shortage of estrogen and testosterone, and cultures, if an infection is suspected.

HOW *NOT* TO TREAT HORMONAL, SYSTEMIC, AND SURGERY-BASED SEXUAL PAIN

Do *not* . . .

- delay treatment.

- avoid or ignore your symptoms.

- feel you are too old to bother.

- avoid treatment for fear of hormonal medications (if carefully planned and followed up on, they are safe).

KEEPING YOUR SEXUAL SIDE ALIVE

Please don't neglect your sexual side during hormonal changes, systemic illness, postoperative recovery, or chemotherapy. Your sexual life is important! We know it can be hard to feel sexually alive when you're going through so much, but the longer you neglect this part of yourself, the harder it will be to resume.

Use this book as your resource, and reach out and get the support you need—from your partner, friends, and whatever professionals or groups you've chosen to help you work through this. Whatever you do, don't decide that your sexual self doesn't matter. It does—and we hope you'll find your own path to sexual recovery and pleasure.

TREATMENTS: WHAT YOU CAN EXPECT

The key thing to remember about treatment for these underlying conditions is that time is of the essence. The longer you're in pain, the more chance that your nerves and muscles will become involved—and in some susceptible women, this can lead to neuropathic pain and pelvic floor dysfunction. If that happens, your pain becomes harder to treat, though it is still treatable.

The first goal of treatment is to protect your delicate vulvar and vaginal tissues, so until therapy begins to take effect, delay attempts at intercourse or penetration for as long as you need to. Follow the genital wellness suggestions given in Chapter 4.

Since fungi (yeast) such as *Candida* are common and easily infect weakened skin, weekly preventative antifungal therapy with oral fluconazole may be needed. We also suggest oral daily probiotic supplements, and, in some cases, vaginal probiotics.

A key treatment goal is to strengthen and increase blood flow to the area. Applying a coating of natural oils like safflower, vitamin E, or olive oil three or four times a day can help your vulvar skin remain hydrated, and in so doing, can actually heal fissures and strengthen it. We've found that compounded low-dose hormones—usually a combination of bioidentical estriol and testosterone—added to these oils have been extremely helpful for strengthening the surface of the vulvar skin and the vestibule. The benefits are usually seen over the course of one or two months.

To lower your pH, strengthen the vaginal mucosa, and rebalance the flora, you might undergo an intravaginal treatment with very low-dose estradiol, estriol, or DHEA capsules. These local medications are safe—even with breastfeeding and in cancer survivors—when used in small doses for the amount of time needed. A daily treatment for two to four weeks followed by a maintenance treatment of once or twice weekly usually suffices.

Many women need systemic testosterone to fully strengthen and heal after their hormonal, systemic, or surgical impacts. Some feel that their lives are restored to normal when they replace this lost hormone. Testosterone transdermal cream helps the low libido and problems with arousal and orgasm that so many women are distressed by during surgical or natural menopause.

Physical therapy is also extremely helpful to treat shortened muscles and connective tissue, and to bring in more blood flow throughout the vulva and pelvis. Home exercise with vaginal dilators is often needed, especially after vaginal surgeries. If accommodating a partner is an issue, you can use a soft donut ring at the vaginal opening to help elongate your canal to receive a penis. Yoga, Pilates, qigong, and other pelvic floor–focused exercises will help immensely after treatment as well, so that you can maintain the gains you have attained.

For some women, systemic hormone therapy—which they may be receiving for other symptoms—will also help the vulva. And if chronic vulvar fissures are unresponsive to the treatments we've described, surgical excision is an option.

SEX AFTER CHEMOTHERAPY

When Lily came to us for consultation, she appeared sad and tired. She told us that a year ago, at age forty-one, she had begun treatment for breast cancer, which was now at an end.

She was relieved but had not been able to even think about resuming intimate contact with her boyfriend. Even to her own touch, her vulvar and vaginal area felt delicate and sore, since her chemotherapy had put her into a menopausal state that would probably persist. She has also had frequent flares of her genital herpes due to her immunological changes.

Lily was at a major loss. Her oncologist had told her that the sexual problems were something she just had to live with, and her gynecologist believed that no topical treatment was safe. Lily felt hopeless—both about her condition and about her relationship.

We reviewed Lily's medical records and told her that the frequent use of hypoallergenic topical oils, like vitamin E and safflower oil, would protect and hydrate her tissues, which might alone be enough for healing. A daily antiviral oral medication, valacyclovir, put the herpes to rest. But Lily, like many women after chemotherapy, also needed the addition of a topical hormonal oil to her vestibule—made of estriol and testosterone, which, when used in very low doses, did wonders.

After only four weeks, Lily's tissues felt normal, and she only needed twice-weekly maintenance therapy with the hormonal oil after that. Her fears evaporated, and she was able to reestablish physical intimacy with her partner.

After having cancer, you may feel doubly ill-fated, finding that now you also have sexual pain. You may not have the mental, physical, and emotional energy yet to focus on healing that pain. We just want you to remember that there is help, and that

➤

> it's worth it for you to take care of yourself in this way—especially since any delay can make the changes more severe and therefore harder to treat.
>
> In many cases, fortifying an intimate relationship or starting a new one may be just what you need to feel like yourself again—which in turn will also help with your long-term healing. Please don't lose hope. It may not seem like it right now, but you will feel more like yourself again with time.

FOR YOUR SEXUAL HEALTH

If you are suffering from the painful sex described in this chapter, always use a lubricant with intercourse or penetration. We recommend that you find a nonirritating brand that works for you. For more on this topic, see the Chapter 14 boxed text "Lubricants Are Our Friends" and the Resources section.

POTENTIAL BREAKTHROUGHS: LOOKING TOWARD THE FUTURE

Research investigating hormones and their relationship to inflammation and neuroinflammation is going on full force. For autoimmune pain, researchers are working with clinicians to move treatments forward.

For example, read what pain management specialist and physiatrist Roberta Shapiro, DO, has to say: "I'm working with a neuroscientist, and she's really the amazing one. I told her the clinical stuff, and she started thinking what she could test for. And we stumbled upon very specific markers that are not done in routine labs—things that absolutely indicate an autoimmune process that has not been identified before."

We have great optimism that progress is coming soon in many fields that will help allay pain in general and sexual pain in particular. (And recently, a new study shows the great benefit of estrogen-lowering medications in preventing breast cancer in high-risk women, meaning many more thousands of women will be offered and treated with these drugs.) Meanwhile, our patients coping with this form of sexual pain are relieved that the treatments they've undergone have made a big difference. But in addition to the medical struggles they've undergone, they also speak of a psychological battle.

"I know there must be millions of women who go through what I went through," says Stephanie. "As terrifying as this is to take on, my message to women is: Don't let your pain go on for years and years. Menopause should not mean an end to your sex life."

PART THREE

OVERCOMING THE PROBLEM

14

REGAINING
SEXUAL JOY

My partner is still very attracted to me, and he does want to have sex, and that makes the situation even harder. Because it doesn't feel good to say no, even if you have to. I feel bad for him and for me. But we are very intimate with each other. We are best friends and hug all the time and are very touchy-feely. We never have stopped that part of our relationship.

—SAVANNAH, REPRODUCTIVE HEALTH WORKER
IN HER EARLY THIRTIES

I am petrified to have sexual intercourse again. All I associate with sex is pain. Also, the only thing now that I associate with my genitals is medical procedures. Although I know that physical therapy is essential for me to get better, it takes away from my sexuality. It is so weird to have people put their fingers in places where you think they never would. . . . What I am saying is that the thought of having anything penetrate that part of my body is only associated with medical procedures and pain. So starting sex sort of feels like another painful chore that I have to do.

—LUCY, FASHION MAGAZINE EDITOR
IN HER LATE TWENTIES

Before this all happened, I was a very healthy person, and I had a good and normal sex life. My libido was fine, and I always enjoyed having sexual contact. I feel something was taken away from me—I feel amputated. I am so sad about this, because I feel blessed with a very good sense of my body, and I came from an intact home, where there were no inhibitions. I feel like the desire is no longer there, and with all the medical tests, I feel like a guinea pig.

—MIRIAM, A HISTORY PROFESSOR IN HER EARLY THIRTIES

As SAVANNAH, LUCY, and Miriam make clear, sexual pain isn't just a physical problem. It affects your sexuality, your relationship, and your entire sense of self. When your intimate parts don't function normally, you can begin to question your entire sense of worth as a woman. No matter how you actually appear to others, or how much reassurance you might receive, when your sexual anatomy is causing you pain, you sometimes feel like the entire world sees you as damaged and undesirable.

According to Dr. Heather Howard, a board-certified sexologist at The Center for Sexual Health and Rehabilitation in San Francisco, "Women suffering from sexual pain also experience a fear of being touched that will lead to sexual escalation, self-doubt, a loss of confidence and trust, feelings of being disadvantaged and victimized, and a disassociation from their bodies." Sexual escalation means that women fear that feelings of sexual satisfaction or an orgasm can exacerbate their pain level.

We've certainly observed this kind of downward spiral in our patients, in which pain, sexual anxiety, and low self-esteem feed on and reinforce each other. This downward spiral can lead to a sense of victimization.

Miriam Biddleman, LCSW, is a well-regarded certified sex therapist in New York City. She says, "I also hear from my patients a lot of 'Why me?' When I treat other patients with medical issues, I don't often hear that. . . . I think women feel this way because they are suffering from a medical anomaly, and because the pain is in such an intimate area. They have never heard of anyone else suffering from this type of pain, and they feel punished. I have a patient who is twenty-nine years old and has multiple sclerosis—and believe it or not, she doesn't feel as bad as women I see with vulvar issues. . . . She doesn't have the shame that women with sexual pain suffer from."

Pain and shame are not the only barriers to sex. It's also hard to feel sexy when you have to put on numerous creams, when you have an ice pack stuck between your legs, when you sense an odor coming from that part of your body, or when you're touching your body not for sexual pleasure but to relieve pain and itching. It's bad enough when sex with another person seems difficult, but even worse when self-pleasuring becomes off-limits.

YOUR ANATOMY DOES NOT DEFINE YOU

What's the solution? You need to begin to redefine your sexuality, so that your sense of yourself as a sexual and sensual woman is not limited by any struggles or frustrations with sexual pain. It is a normal reaction to feel desexualized by your pain, and by all the exams and procedures you must endure to get better. And we are not saying that it's easy to reframe the way you think about your sexuality. But it is essential not to equate typically functioning anatomical parts with sensuality and sexuality. There is so much more that makes you a vibrant and sexual woman.

When pain makes it impossible to have intercourse, many women share how much they desperately miss the intimate experience involved with this part of sex. At a recent medical conference on endometriosis, women suffering from sexual pain spoke about how intercourse provides more than intimacy with a partner—how it is actually, for many women, a spiritual and transcendental experience. Some also said that, for them, no other form of sexual intimacy induces the same level of connectedness or union with another being.

We understand that for many of you, sexual intercourse is your ultimate goal, and we hope that our recommendations and your medical and psychological journey will help you attain this. However, until you are able to physically tolerate sexual penetration, we would like to help you find ways to achieve sexual satisfaction and intimacy in your relationships. Most importantly, do not give up on other sexual activities just because you cannot have intercourse. Remaining intimate will physically and emotionally strengthen you, and will better allow you to achieve your goal of intercourse when you are ready.

REFRAMING YOUR THOUGHTS

It isn't easy, but it is possible to change the way you think by using a common cognitive-behavioral technique known as "thought stopping" or "thought reprogramming." If you commit to practicing this technique, eventually, your heart will start to believe what your mind initiates. The process is neither automatic nor easy, but it can be learned. Here's what to do.

Whenever you find yourself thinking a negative thought about yourself, your body, or your sexuality, take note. Then force yourself to interrupt the thought and replace it with a positive thought. If necessary, make a list of positive thoughts, or choose a single reliable thought. Here are some examples:

- "My sensuality and sexuality are defined by so many parts of my personality, including my sense of humor, intelligence, and creativity."

- "I love myself and my body because of who I am as a person, not because of my genitals."

- "I don't always feel like having sex, but I am still a vibrant and sexual woman."

➤

> The key is to ask your mind to affirm this view of yourself, even if it's not how you happen to feel at the moment. If you rigorously practice this technique, your rewritten thoughts will lead to new feelings and a renewed self-image.
>
> If you need help practicing, there are many well-trained psychotherapists who can help you. Many women also find that yoga or meditation helps them clear their minds of negative thoughts and perceptions.
>
> One final word: Don't worry if some days you are just not up to practicing this technique. Let yourself have ups and downs. Just commit to doing the best you can, and keep practicing.

PAIN, INTIMACY, AND DESIRE

Pain usually makes you feel less sexy—and that goes triple for sexual pain. A sad byproduct of this natural response is that the resulting lack of sex often affects the level of intimacy in a relationship. Just as sexual pain can snowball into low self-esteem, the fear of sexual pain can turn into hypervigilance, anxiety, and depression—all of which can make you feel even more detached from your partner.

Even after your sexual pain has been resolved, you might feel a distinct loss in libido and desire especially when sexual activity becomes mentally associated with pain. If you're in a committed relationship, your partner's libido may also have declined, because he or she also associates sex with causing you pain.

Miriam, quoted at the beginning of this chapter, felt a loss of libido, even after her sexual pain had been healed. Lynn, a retired teacher in her late fifties, had a similar loss of libido. She is now able to have intercourse with her husband as long as he is very careful not to touch parts that are very sensitive. "But for a long time," she says, "I felt nothing sexually. And that was really bad for me, especially because I am a very sensual woman. I like to look and dress sexy and flirt—and for a good number of years when this started, I felt like a nonentity. I didn't feel like a woman at all, and that stress and depression made the pain even worse."

Lynn was clear, however, that these responses were hers and not her partner's. "My husband never made me feel like that," she says. "He always thought of me as a sexy woman, whether I could have sex or not. He has been great throughout all of these years, but it was in my own head—and that made me even more miserable."

If you're feeling a loss of libido, you may be responding to continuing pain or to memories of pain. But you may also be responding to the stress of everything you've been through. Ironically, when many men feel stressed, they may respond by wanting sex more, as a kind of stress reducer. For many women, though, stress erodes desire. So even as you're feeling better physically, stress may make it harder to feel sexy again.

Another factor in your sexual desire might be medical. If your doctor has prescribed antidepressants or antianxiety medications, you may be experiencing the well-documented side effect of "decreased libido." SSRIs such as fluoxetine (Prozac), citalopram (Celexa), and sertraline (Zoloft), or SNRIs such as bupropion (Wellbutrin), venlafaxine (Effexor), duloxetine (Cymbalta), and milnacipran (Savella), may be reducing your desire, as might such anticonvulsants as gabapentin (Neurontin) and pregabalin (Lyrica).

Many of these medications also add to your fatigue, which further undermines your libido, and cause constipation, adding to discomfort. Speak to your doctor about a change in medications or about the addition of testosterone or DHEA, or another medication that might improve your libido.

FEELING SEXY AGAIN

Our patients feel sexy when they treat themselves well. If you feel like you've lost your sexual sparkle, consider one of the following morale boosters:

- buy a sexy new dress, lingerie, or shoes;

- get a new hairstyle or color;

- watch romantic and sexy movies, or read romantic novels;

- exercise and watch yourself improve;

- get some new makeup, a manicure, or a pedicure;

- go for a massage or spa treatment; or

- fantasize and masturbate.

Appreciate your feelings of sexiness when they come up—enjoy them, and don't push them away.

INTIMACY AND YOUR PARTNER

Even while you're struggling with your own sexual issues, your partner may be having similar concerns. Many men respond to a partner's sexual pain by becoming impotent, resulting from the belief (irrational as it may be) that he is at fault for your sexual pain or that he is a failed man for not being able to help you.

Besides a partner's sexual pain, a man may be struggling with other sexual issues, which are surprisingly common. Among men who have reached the age of forty, some 30 percent have hypoactive sexual desire disorder (low libido); 30 percent have various degrees of orgasmic dysfunction; and 10 percent have erectile dysfunction. If your partner has the added worry that he may hurt you while having sex, he may be even more likely to struggle with sexual dysfunction.

When a man perceives that his responses are making things more difficult for the woman he loves, he may withdraw or shut down emotionally, become angry, become more insistent sexually, or compensate in some other way. This in turn makes you feel worse, and perhaps you withdraw, respond with anger, or otherwise interrupt your intimacy. The two of you may still care deeply for each other—but you may also feel a significant distance, emotionally as well as sexually.

Our patient Stephanie experienced particular difficulties with this cycle. "My husband physically and emotionally disconnected himself from me and was angry at me for not being able to have intercourse," she says. "He was not supportive at all. He felt like sex was an all or nothing deal—it's either intercourse or nothing. Of course he would give me a kiss here and there but would not do anything else."

Stephanie felt deeply disturbed by her partner's reactions. "His attitude was so disturbing to me," she says. "I used to weep about it all the time. And his anger at me perpetuated a whole vicious cycle and instilled a great deal of anger in me toward him. He felt deprived and miserable—he recognized that I couldn't help the pain, but he felt like it was my problem. . . . I was so angry at him for what I thought was a very narrow-minded view about lovemaking. . . . I felt guilty, sad, and depressed most of the time."

Though life at home was terrible, her work life still gave her intellectual and ego gratification. Although work was essential, Stephanie could never totally escape her feelings of inadequacy as a woman. "I functioned at work very well, and no one knew the physical and emotional pain that I endured. At times I don't know how my marriage lasted, because it was just so hard. I felt so alone and betrayed. There was basically no intimacy in our marriage, even though my husband and I love each other very much."

Luckily, Stephanie was able to recover from her sexual pain with physical therapy and the medical treatments that Deborah provided. Being able to have intercourse with her husband made an enormous difference in their relationship. "We have had sexual intercourse twice already," she says. "The first time was a little awkward and painful, and the second time was a little better. I wouldn't say orgasms were flying here and there, but I felt so much better, and felt a great deal of relief and hope. . . . And my husband has been much more kissy-friendly, and he puts his arms around me at night."

Stephanie's sexual recovery enabled her marital recovery, but not every woman is so lucky. Many of our patients have a harder road back from the loss of intimacy brought about by sexual pain. That's why so many sexual-health professionals recommend couples therapy when a woman struggles with sexual pain. Our colleague Kristene Whitmore, MD, medical director of the Pelvic and Sexual Health Institute in Philadelphia, goes so far as to call couples therapy "essential."

SEXUAL HEALING

Once the sexual pain has begun to recede, how do you regain your sexual joy? Like every other type of healing, sexual recovery is a process involving mind, body, spirit—and a lot of patience. Whether you're in a committed relationship, a newer relationship, or single, you can make your way back to a place of sexual pleasure and intimacy. It may take a while, and you may have some setbacks along the way, but please don't give up. Sexual healing and renewed intimacy are possible for you, we promise.

Restoring Your Body

To begin your healing journey, do everything you can to support your physical health. You might want to look back to Chapter 4 for our recommendations on how to support your nutrition, sleep, and well-being. Yoga, meditation, qigong, tai chi, Pilates, hypnosis and self-hypnosis, and acupuncture can all be extremely helpful—as can guided imagery and other types of cognitive–behavioral techniques. We repeat our recommendation for working with a therapist who understands both sexual recovery and chronic pain.

We also can't stress too strongly the importance of good, restful sleep. Many studies show that poor sleep decreases libido, especially during and after menopause. One of the best things you can do for your sex life is to make sure you are getting enough deep sleep.

Herbal and Medicinal Aids

Testosterone supplements may help restore your libido. Talk with your healthcare practitioner about the possibility of using testosterone cream, which you can apply to your skin. In one study, 60 to 70 percent of the women using testosterone experienced an increased libido within about six to eight weeks.

Another support for libido is the natural herbal product Arginmax, which might take one or two months to work. This supplement is not for women with high blood pressure and some other health conditions, so if you're considering taking it, make sure to check with your doctor.

Achieving Calm

One of the worst aftereffects of sexual pain is the fear of its return—and the related anxiety that might attach to anything that seems to even remotely signal a potential problem.

For example, one of Deborah's patients assumed that if she had bladder leakage while doing aerobics, she would also leak during sex. The possibility upset her so much that she avoided dating altogether. Fortunately, Deborah was able to reassure her that there was no connection whatsoever between what took place during exercise and what might happen during sex, but coping with such disturbing thoughts and persistent fears is often part of recovery.

If you find yourself fearful, hypervigilant, anxious, or prone to think the worst, we urge you to work with a therapist trained in cognitive–behavioral techniques who can help you repattern your thoughts and therefore feel calmer. Again, yoga, meditation, and other modalities discussed in Chapter 4 can help you feel calmer as well.

IF YOU'RE SINGLE

We have enormous sympathy for the difficulties of starting to date during or after a struggle with sexual pain. We know that it's not easy to open up to a new person in your life while so much else is going on, and that even after you've recovered physically, you may feel anxious, discouraged, or simply numb when it comes to "getting out there" again.

Perhaps you've taken yourself out of the dating pool for fear of no longer being desirable. Or maybe you dread the idea of having to explain your condition to someone.

As a single woman dealing with sexual pain, you do face additional obstacles that women who are in committed relationships don't have to face. However, the pain doesn't have to put an end to your romantic life. You may not want to open yourself up that way for only casual sex, but certainly, with someone you care for, it's worth finding out what the possibilities are.

The key is not to define your sexuality by how your intimate parts function—and then not to allow a potential partner to define you that way either. If another person finds you attractive, then the two of you can find ways to make each other happy, even if you have to be more creative sexually. Remember, no person is attracted to you just because of your vulva and vagina. If they're interested, they're interested in the whole package.

Talking about Sex with a Potential Partner

If you want to tell a potential romantic partner about your sexual pain, here are some ways to approach it:

I really enjoy sex, but I have a condition that affects me physically, and that sometimes causes me pain during sex. We can definitely get there—but we'll have to take it slow.

I have a condition that means I shouldn't have intercourse, at least not until I'm better. I'm working with a great doctor, and things are very hopeful. Meanwhile, what I've learned from this experience is that there are lots of ways to get creative sexually. Then, when we can have intercourse, we'll have that creative stuff and the regular stuff!

I have a condition that affects what I can do sexually, because sex and intimate touch cause me a lot of pain. I don't have an STD, and what I have is not contagious, but it is a physical condition—it's not psychological. I can enjoy being sexual with you, and my ultimate goal is to be able to have intercourse, but that may take quite a while. Meanwhile, we'll just have to figure out where you can touch me, and where I can touch you—and how we can make each other happy.

Your condition might mean that you and your partner will need to wait longer to have sex than you otherwise would, and that the two of you will have to make more allowances for what works for you. Again, in a casual relationship, this might be asking too much—but in any relationship that's based on mutual caring rather than simply the desire for sex, both people will expect to make sacrifices and compromises. If someone rejects you because of your sexual pain, you probably wouldn't want to be in a relationship with that person anyway.

KELSEY'S STORY

Kelsey, age twenty-seven, is a successful marketing executive for a designer clothing manufacturer. For the past two years, she has had a loving boyfriend. But because she was diagnosed before she was ever sexually active, her struggles with sexual pain shaped her entire first experience of sex.

>

"I was devastated that I never experienced sex as a normal and healthy person," Kelsey says. "I dated one guy in college, and when I told him about my problem, he totally freaked out and never spoke to me again. . . . I told him I didn't have an STD, and that I have pelvic pain and am being treated by a doctor and will get better. But he never talked to me again and defriended me on Facebook. Who does that?"

In general, dating in college was extremely challenging. "It was really hard in college because I did go to bars, but all I could do was kiss, and that wasn't really acceptable to guys," says Kelsey. "In college, you kiss like two times and then you have to move onto something else. I didn't know what to do. So I didn't end up having a boyfriend in college, and I think I might have acted differently around guys, because in the back of my head, I knew I could only go so far."

But things turned around for her. "I did finally have one boyfriend who was great about my condition. Then, after we broke up, a half a year later, I met another guy at a party, and we have been together for more than two years. He has been unbelievably understanding about my sexual pain. It was very surprising to me, because he was a frat guy in college, and I think he dated a lot of girls. But he has been so supportive of me throughout all my treatments and surgery."

Her physical therapist also offered a good deal of emotional support. Kelsey remembers, "My physical therapist said to me 'You will find a guy who will like you for you.' And when I met my boyfriend, I finally realized she was right. If a guy rejects you because of your sexual-pain issue, then he is not worth being with anyway."

After she had been seeing her current boyfriend for a year and a half, Kelsey finally had a vestibulectomy, which helped a lot. But she still struggles with sexual pain.

"After sex, it takes me about a day to feel better," she says. "There are times when I say to my boyfriend that I can't have sex, and I feel bad about it. But neither of us wants me to be in pain. There was one time I started crying, and he immediately pulled back, because he didn't want to hurt me. . . . I think we have found a way to keep our intimacy. He knows what's uncomfortable for me, and if I say something is uncomfortable, he backs off, so I never feel pressured. He also loves cuddling, and he said he never did that before me. I think we really have a good bond. My boyfriend says to me often that we've gone through a lot, and 'I am definitely in this with you for the long haul.'"

Kelsey's story is inspiring: It shows that dating and a growing intimacy are possible, even when you struggle with sexual pain. Developing a relationship under these conditions may be a challenge, but it can be done—and the final result may well make all the hard work worthwhile.

IF YOU'RE IN A COMMITTED RELATIONSHIP

Within a committed relationship, there are two issues: your libido and your intimacy. Once you're able to restore your sense of yourself as a sexual, desirable woman, you may find that your libido begins to rise. As you become more relaxed and more sexually interested, your partner's libido may return as well.

Wherever you and your partner are sexually, it's crucial for the two of you to remain intimate in as many ways as possible. Communicating with your partner is very helpful in restoring closeness.

Please don't ever pressure yourself into having any type of sexual activity, especially if you're having a really painful day or a flare-up. We're not opposed to sometimes accommodating your partner, but not if you're in too much pain to even be touched. You need to let your partner know what's going on, so he or she doesn't feel rejected.

Miriam Biddleman has some terrific advice for women reentering the sexual arena:

> *I have to explain to patients that they have to pace themselves sexually. It is a very scary thing to begin any kind of sexual activity. Women who have had sexual pain for a long time have a hard time determining what is "normal." It is important to tell patients that everyone's "normal" is different—that there is no right or wrong. And women and their partners need to go at their own pace; no one should push themselves.*

You also need to remember that although your partner isn't feeling your physical pain, he or she is experiencing profound trauma, because it's hard for them to see you in such horrendous pain and feel so powerless to help. It's even harder for them to feel that they are at least partly the cause of your distress. Recognizing your partner's feelings while he or she recognizes yours is a wonderful basis for reigniting both passion and intimacy.

If You're Partnered with a Man

Often, male partners want to fix a situation, when women merely want to be able to vent and receive emotional support. You can tell your partner that you are not looking for solutions; that you just want someone to recognize your feelings, to lend a supportive ear, give a warm hug, and offer reassurance. This form of communication alone can renew closeness and intimacy.

It's also important for you to be able to hear your partner's feelings and concerns. Many men are not comfortable sharing their feelings, but if you have a male partner, encourage him to speak as freely as he can, and affirm you are able to emotionally handle any feelings he might be going through—including fears for the future, anger at you for bringing this problem into his life, and doubts about his own sexuality. It can be very frightening for a man to feel that his sexual needs literally cause pain to the woman he loves, and many men react to that by feeling as though their own sexuality were some-how defective. Other men have trouble feeling confident in their sexuality if they're not actually having intercourse.

Even when a relationship is close, the process of reestablishing intimacy can be tricky. "I once spoke with my husband about our inability to have sex, and I told him he could have an affair, because this was not about him," admits Kate. "I felt tremendous guilt about not being able to have sex with him. But I never felt sexually inadequate. Sexually I feel good about myself, and very intact."

"I can be intimate with my husband at times," says Lynn. "We do have intercourse occasionally, and he is always concerned that he is hurting me. But because I'm in pain all the time, I'm not often in the mood. . . . One act of intimacy that I do miss is our laughing together in bed. We don't always sleep in the same bed because of his snoring. But when we do sleep together, and talk and laugh the way we used to, I feel so much closer to him and feel a strong sense of intimacy. We don't need sex to feel intimacy."

BETH'S STORY

"The intimacy between my husband and me was severely affected," says Beth, a freelance writer in her late forties. "He was incredibly supportive during my entire illness, and never made me feel like I was exaggerating my symptoms. He knew what a strong person I was. But we didn't touch each other enough or find other ways to be intimate with each other, because we were so drained and debilitated by my physical and our emotional pain.

"We are now working to regain some level of intimacy, but it is not an easy road. It is something we really have to work at, with determination and perseverance. It's not that our love for

➤

each other has been compromised—in fact, I feel like it's stronger than ever. It's just that having such a serious illness that affected the core of my sexual identity really took a tremendous toll on the level of physical intimacy in our life. We can have sex without pain. But I feel like my husband's libido was greatly affected by my illness. I feel like, as a matter of self-preservation, he had to shut down, and we are slowly trying to open up his libido valve. It is hard for me not to take it personally, but we really had to sit down and talk about how his physical withdrawal from me was making me feel. I told him I was feeling rejected, and that I was being doubly punished for having an illness that affected my vulva. Not only was my sexual identity so compromised, but I was being rejected due to this illness. I told him how unfair I felt he was being, but I also told him I understood what an emotional toll this took on him sexually.

"It will take a lot of time, patience, and work to regain a sex life—and who knows how much of a sex life we will ever have? I think this illness took a permanent toll on our sex life. But even if we don't ever return to what we had before, I can live with that. But we will constantly have to work at this."

For Beth and her husband, couples therapy was crucial in reestablishing intimacy. "My husband and I could not have gotten through this ordeal without couples therapy," she says. "During our last session, my husband shared with me that when I don't share how much pain I am in, he feels very distant from me, because I act different, and he doesn't know what is going on with me. I, on the other hand, try to protect him, and I feel he is so tired of hearing about my pain, so I hide how much pain I am in.

"I was very proud of him, because he really shared his feelings, and I didn't feel attacked. What this showed me—with the help of a very skilled therapist—is that I need to be honest

> and communicate with him all the time. If I don't, then I create a distance between us, and our intimacy suffers. I was totally unaware I was doing this. That session alone greatly increased our intimacy. Even the best sex couldn't have made me feel closer to my husband. So I learned that a partner who really cares about you *wants* to know about your pain, and I cannot protect him from my pain. Our relationship suffers when I get too stoic.
>
> "I also learned that true intimacy is not dependent on sexual intercourse—it's a real sharing of your self. I know that may sound corny, but it's true."

If You're Partnered with a Woman

Possibly, because you share the same anatomy, your partner may be more easily able to empathize with your pain. But by the same token, she may overidentify with your condition or fear developing it herself, without some of the boundaries that heterosexual partners can take for granted. You and your partner may need to work on these kinds of boundaries as you continue your healing journey.

JazzE, a fifty-year-old woman with painful bladder syndrome, has been with her current partner for two years. She admits, "I don't like to share my sexual-pain problems with my partner. . . . But my partner is wonderful, and I know she would totally understand my sexual pain. It's my problem that I don't share my concerns, not hers. I have had a lot of medical issues, and I don't want to burden her with another issue."

Though JazzE chooses not to talk about her pain, she has found a way to have a fulfilling sex life with her partner. "Because of my sexual-pain issues, I often don't want her to touch me in the vulvovaginal area. I want to be the one touching—I want to be the aggressor. In my world, it's called being a stone dyke: It's where you want to do all the touching and pleasuring, and you feel fine not being touched or pleasured. I don't need to be touched in the vaginal region. But I love being touched in all other areas of my body. We have a very intimate relationship. I love cuddling and even oral sex," she says.

"Overall, my relationship with my partner is beautiful. And it is that way because we are both very warm, loving, and nurturing."

Talking about Sex with Your Partner

Talking about sex can also be helpful, even if it's uncomfortable. You might want to plan what you want to say, or even write down some thoughts. The conversation may well include a discussion of new sexual activities, so it's okay to laugh and feel a little embarrassed.

Once the conversation begins, try not to interrupt your partner. Also, try not to tell your partner how she or he thinks or feels. All responses in this situation are valid, even if you don't agree with each other.

Here are some specific tips about how to talk about sex issues with your partner. Some may be appropriate for your situation, some not.

- Talk about what you enjoyed in your sex life before sexual pain began.

- Explain how sexual pain has changed your experience of sex.

- Encourage your partner to be honest about his or her feelings.

- Tell your partner exactly which kinds of touch hurt and which areas of your vulva and pelvis you prefer not be touched.

- Tell your partner exactly which kinds of touch give you pleasure, and which kinds of positions and sexual acts you enjoy.

- Explain which kinds of nonsexual gestures make you feel loved and valued—such as attending doctor's visits with you, holding your hand, scratching your back, asking you out on a date, giving you a card, calling during the day to ask how you are feeling, or bringing you flowers.

• Ask your partner what you can do for them to make them feel loved and valued, especially at times when you are not able to be sexually intimate.

• Invite your partner to come with you to a medical or physical therapy appointment so a professional can show exactly where you're sensitive and can answer any questions he or she may have about your condition.

LUBRICANTS ARE OUR FRIENDS

One of the things that can make sexual contact much, much easier is finding the right lubricant. When you're well lubricated, you're far more likely to find being touched sensual and exciting. (If you want to test this theory, try running your finger over your lips when they're dry, and then doing the same thing when you've moistened your lips. Notice the difference in sensation?)

The right lubricant is the one that doesn't irritate and exacerbate any ongoing or residual sexual discomfort—especially if you have skin pain. If you're not using condoms, you can use a wide variety of natural, gentle oils: olive, almond, safflower, or coconut. Water-based lubricants have the fewest ingredients and work very well, but silicone-based ones last longer if that is what you need. Some recommended over-the-counter lubricants include Slippery Stuff, FemGlide, and Glide. Natural lubricants include saliva and egg white. Many women prefer long-acting vaginal moisturizers such as Replens, which, if used regularly every 2-4 days, helps vaginal dryness without adding

>

➤ estrogen (as has been studied in women with breast cancer). A good lubricant for couples trying to conceive is called Pre-Seed, which is also well liked for general use.

Please avoid glycerin or spermicidal lubricants, which are quite irritating, and never use them anally. Avoid anything anti-bacterial or containing a soap, perfume, or preservatives. Avoid products that don't include a list of ingredients.

When using a lubricant, just spread a thin layer on the genital surfaces of both partners, add a little extra at the posterior fourchette (see illustration 6-1 in Chapter 6), and remember to repeat this as needed.

REDEFINING SEX

If you're going to re-create your sex life during or after a sexual-pain condition, we invite you to broaden your view of what defines sex. Like many women with pelvic or vulvar pain, you might not be able to have sexual intercourse for some time—perhaps for a very long time. But you are still a sexual being who can engage in joyful sexual acts.

We like what Miriam Biddleman has to say about sex.

Sex is between our ears. Sexuality is an energy; it includes any activity that attracts us, that warms us, that feels healing and loving. When you give and receive sexual pleasure, you are having sex, it doesn't matter how.

Redefining the Role of Orgasm

Here's Ms. Biddleman again:

When I was growing up, sex meant everything. It meant foreplay, kissing, oral sex—whatever gave you sexual pleasure, from cuddling to snuggling. I've come to learn now that when people say "sex," they mean "intercourse." So what I come up against a lot is: "The gold standard is intercourse with orgasms."

Sex is a banquet. . . . sex is a smorgasbord. There are so many things that you can do that are not only sexual but also arousing—things that don't have to do with sticking anything up your vagina or with wild pounding sex. When I speak with patients, I talk about a variety of activities that they can do that are extremely intimate—including spooning and synchronicity of breathing. It's not orgasm; it's just tremendous intimacy, closeness, and a lot of touching. It's a reeducation of what arousal can be.

Pioneering sex researcher Beverly Whipple, PhD, RN, FAAN, suggests that instead of thinking of orgasm as our ultimate goal, we should emphasize "pleasure-directed sexuality." In other words, we should not think of an orgasm as something to attain but instead as something that may or may not be experienced while engaging in pleasurable sexual activity.

Likewise, sex therapists Masters and Johnson suggest that couples who are resuming sexual activity after a long dry spell work toward a "sensate focus"—a focus on savoring the senses—rather than only on achieving orgasm.

Tantric Sex

Believed to date back five thousand years, tantra is an ancient esoteric practice in which expanded orgasm is considered to be a direct path to spiritual enlightenment. In the West, even those who don't practice Eastern religions have incorporated many tantric sexual techniques in a quest for sexual pleasure. Since tantric sex is based on using nonpenetrative ways to induce orgasm, it can be a wonderful practice while going through or recovering from sexual pain.

The key to tantric sex is breath. If you can keep your body relaxed and your mind clear of the mundane (which we realize may be quite a challenge!), you can become more fully present.

Orgasm and penetration are not the main objectives of tantric sex. Instead, you attempt to prolong the act, increasing potent sexual energy and intimacy with your partner. If you focus only on the "final act" of sex, you miss the amazing range of feelings the rest of sex has to offer.

Here are some basic tantric techniques you can try out:

Create an intimate space.

This should be a comfortable area that is playful and relaxed. It doesn't have to be your bedroom—just find a space where you can feel at ease. You can play music or have scented candles—use anything that will make your space feel romantic.

Don't pressure yourself.

Go as slowly as you need to. Keep in mind that this might feel very unnatural and even a little goofy to you at first—especially if you have stayed away from any sexual activity for a while due to your pain.

Be aware of each other's breathing.

Watching your partner's breathing and trying to be in sync with each other's breathing can be a very intimate action. Sit close to each other, and inhale while your partner exhales and vice versa. As your partner breathes out, you'll find yourself taking their breath into and down through your entire body. In this way, you are sharing all of yourself with your partner. Becoming conscious about your breath is central to all yoga practices and is essential in tantra.

Pace yourself.

Foreplay is essential in tantra. However, we are not going to refer to your activity as foreplay, because the goal of your sexual actions may not be orgasm and most likely is not penetration. All the activities in which you might engage—mutual masturbation, cuddling, oral sex, spooning, hand holding, or caressing—should be done slowly. If you don't become aroused, don't worry. Arousal and orgasm may or may not be your goals. Please don't panic or worry that you never will be at that point again. The goal right now is intimacy.

WAYS TO FEEL SEXIER WITH YOUR PARTNER

- Hold hands while walking, watching TV, or sitting in a movie theater.

- When you're up to it, go on a date.

- Make sure to talk in a quiet, relaxed setting for at least twenty minutes every few days.

- Give each other special presents.

- Learn how to give each other massages—or, if sexual pain and/or back issues make that problematic, learn how to give each other foot massages.

- Share a favorite activity.

- Find a way to laugh together—a comedy show, a funny movie, a visit with a friend who makes you laugh, a conversation about something you both find funny.

- Share a sexual fantasy.

- Play with the sexiness of one person doing all the touching and the other person receiving all the touch (but be sure to switch roles!).

- Take turns playfully "commanding" each other to perform different sexual acts.

➤

- Find sexy ways to touch parts of the body that are not part of the pelvis.

- Shop together for sex toys—or you can each choose one in secret and surprise your partner with it.

- Explore the sensual possibilities of a feather, a piece of silk, a piece of fur, and other tactile objects.

WHEN THE PAIN IS GONE

Even if a woman has completely recovered from sexual pain, there are still residual emotional ramifications that affect renewing a sexual relationship. Women who have recovered from sexual pain can still suffer psychological trauma and may not be eager to resume an active sexual relationship. As we have seen, living with sexual pain for a long time can diminish your libido significantly. Reigniting your libido may take a great deal of time and effort. It doesn't turn back on automatically once the pain is gone.

The most important thing you can do at this stage of your recovery is to give yourself time and to be patient with yourself and your partner, who may be hesitant to resume sexual intercourse out of fear of hurting you.

It is normal to be anxious about having sexual intercourse, even if you are given the green light by your doctor. As with any trauma or loss, it takes time to emotionally recover and gain your confidence and bearings. You have been through a horrendous physical and emotional ordeal, and as with anyone who has suffered from a serious medical condition, you might feel anxiety and fear.

We advise you not to have too many expectations the first few times you try to have intercourse. Don't expect bells to be ringing and fireworks to be flaring. (Remember that in even the very best of circumstances, committed couples only rate 40 percent of sexual events between them as "good" for both!) You should try to make yourselves as relaxed as possible, but expect that you might be anxious and nervous the first few times you try. You might also want to use a lubricant to help ease intercourse. (See the boxed text.) Many patients who have pelvic floor tightness have found that vaginal diazepam (Valium) tablets placed two hours before sexual activity can be helpful. Also, using vaginal dilators during foreplay, with your partner's participation, may help. Speak to your physical therapist about the many techniques that can ease intercourse.

What you most likely will see after time is that intercourse will become more natural and more enjoyable. Even if intercourse produces some discomfort, remember you have not had anything penetrate your vagina for quite a long time, so any friction may be initially irritating.

But just as with any emotional recovery, there is no time limit or timeline you should follow. However long it takes you to get comfortable is natural and normal. You may not ever resume the same level of activity that you had prior to your medical condition—or you may have an even more active sex life.

Be patient with yourself, be open, and don't be judgmental of yourself or your partner. You have done a remarkable job dealing with all aspects of your condition, and you should be exceedingly proud of yourself. It's as if you have visited a foreign planet without the proper navigation equipment, but still found a way to navigate your journey back with courage, creativity, humor, and perseverance.

We'd like to leave you with the conclusion of our conversation with our patient Lucy. "Is there any way that intercourse might be fun for me and my boyfriend the first time?" she asked us.

We explained that Lucy's first few times might be a little irritating, but we felt certain that in time, she and her boyfriend would be able once again to resume a gratifying, fun, and joyful sex life. For the first time, a smile began to appear on Lucy's face.

15

· · · · · · · · ·

HEALING

YOUR

RELATIONSHIPS

"I worry that my friends are tired of hearing about how sick I am."

*"I don't know how to explain all my absences at work. My cowork-
ers are getting tired of having to cover for me when they don't
even know what's wrong."*

*"My family knows I have some kind of medical problem, but they
don't know the details—and I don't want them to know."*

*"I think it's been hard on my kids, seeing Mommy be sick so often.
I haven't figured out how to explain it to them, or how to tell
them not to worry."*

*"My husband and I have started having sex again. But we haven't
figured out how to get back to the way we were."*

*"My significant other was really shaken up by all this—seeing me
sick, seeing me in pain. I'm not sure how we're going to work it
all out."*

W E KNOW THAT sexual pain can take a toll on all your relationships including those with your partner, family members, coworkers, employers, and friends. This chapter addresses how your pain may affect your relationships and gives you the necessary tools to mend and heal the stressed connections with the people most important to you.

Sexual pain doesn't just take its toll on your body, your spirits, and your libido. It also has a profound effect on your relationships. When the pain is at its worst and you feel as if you can barely survive, you may not have even a spare ounce of energy to think about anything but how to make it through the next five minutes. But when you do have some breathing room, you will be ready to give your relationships some attention.

Finding the balance between yourself and your relationships is hard for many women. Many of us tend to pour ourselves into partner, children, friends, and work, with little energy or care left over for ourselves. When crisis strikes, it can be even harder to right the balance—to make time for ourselves while also keeping precious relationships alive. The problem is all the more complicated because we need our relationships for emotional support and to help keep us sane.

MAINTAINING RELATIONSHIPS

Here are a few suggestions for how to maintain relationships while you're struggling with sexual pain.

Make your own decisions about who you're going to tell and how much you'll share.

The important thing to remember is that your decisions don't have to be "all or nothing." Letting important people in your life know at least something about what's going on (rather than shutting them out completely) may enable you to feel closer to them—and it may make it easier for them to feel closer to you, and to be there for you in ways you will appreciate. Here is one way you might share information while setting boundaries.

I'm struggling with a medical problem at the moment. It's not life-threatening, so you don't have to worry, but I am often in a lot of pain. I'd really rather not talk about the details, but you're important to me, and I wanted you to know. If I drop out of sight for a bit or seem unavailable for some of the things we usually do together, it might be that I'm having treatments or am in pain, and I hope you won't take it personally. I really appreciate knowing you're there—and thanks for letting me keep this private.

Be as clear as you can about what you would like the other person to do.

One of the hardest parts of seeing someone you care for in pain—whether emotional or physical pain—is not knowing when to reach out and when to pull back. If you can cue your people about your wishes, both they and you will be more comfortable—and you're more likely to get what you want. Here are some suggestions:

"It makes me feel great when you ask how I am. I'll probably give you a general answer without any medical details, but I love knowing you're concerned."

"Please don't ask me how I am. If I want to talk about my condition, I'll bring it up, but sometimes I just want a break from thinking about it and talking about it. I love that you're concerned—but I'd be so grateful if you'd let me be the one to bring it up."

"I really appreciate your calling and asking me to do things, even if so much of the time I have to say no. Would you be willing to keep calling, and not take it personally if I say no? It would mean so much to me."

"It's so nice of you to keep calling—but I feel so bad having to say no all the time. Would it be okay if you let me be the one to initiate getting together? This is just such a hard time—I really appreciate your letting me be the one to think about socializing or not."

"It actually doesn't work for me when you do [something you don't like], but it would be wonderful if you would do [something you do like]."

"Please don't be hurt if I don't always answer the phone or your emails; sometimes I am too exhausted or in too much pain to talk or to sit and type. But hearing your messages of support on my answering machine and receiving your emails means the world to me."

In all these suggestions, you can see how we've steered you toward affirming how important the other person is to you and how much their presence means in your life. Tell the people closest to you how grateful you are for their support. Give the message of what you want while also conveying your feelings about the person and the relationship.

Things change, so check in with yourself periodically.

What you wanted the day you got your diagnosis isn't necessarily the same as what you want two weeks, two months, or two years in. You and your situation keep changing, and what you want from the important people in your life will probably change as well, almost certainly more than once. If you do decide to make new decisions—to start socializing after a period of isolation, or to withdraw a bit after a period of being more in touch—do your best to communicate this decision to your loved ones. And again, be as clear as you can about what you want from them.

Be creative about how to stay in touch.

Sometimes it's exhausting to talk to people in person or even on the phone, especially if you're in pain or feeling tired and discouraged. Get creative. Ask a loved one to pass the news on to other friends and family; write a mass email that is shared among your loved ones; or come up with your own idea of the kind of contact that is perfect for you: "Come and do errands with me!" "I have to take a walk each morning anyway; can you join me one day and walk with me?" "Maybe you could give me a lift to the hairdresser? At least we'd have the fifteen minutes in the car." Sometimes even a little contact is better than none, and the relationship will then be easier to resume when you're feeling better.

Be as generous as you can stand to be about your loved ones'
limitations.

Even the most understanding people in your life cannot totally grasp the enormity of the pain you are experiencing. People with other types of pain conditions—such as those dealing with backaches and migraines—may try to empathize with your pain, but what you're feeling may very well be more intense, more severe, and more intimately bound up with your identity. Do what you can to make allowances for people who simply don't understand what you're going through—although it's also fine to ask them not to draw the comparison and not to give you advice.

EXPLAINING YOUR CONDITION TO FRIENDS AND FAMILY

We know you don't need another job at this point, but if you want support from family and friends, your job is to educate people about your medical condition. You also need to tell people that your reactions to this often agonizing pain are normal. Explain that what you need from your loved ones is compassion, empathy, and validation of your feelings—not false reassurance, advice, or stories about similar conditions that they or someone else has experienced.

Beth shared how she told family and friends about her situation. "I feel very lucky to have such a supportive family and friends," she says. "They all know that I am not a complainer and that I am pretty stoic. So when I told them about how agonizing my pain was, they really seemed to get it. I told my sister and a select group of friends, and when I had rough days or needed help, it was so helpful to know that they didn't expect me to act the way I normally did. I feel like it took a lot of pressure off of me."

Nicole, a fulltime mother in her mid-thirties with a labral tear in her hip, told us that she didn't want to tell her friends about her pain. "I didn't want it to become my identity," she says. She did tell her mother and sister, but says, "I know they feel so helpless and don't always know what to say to me."

Lynn, who is suffering from central nervous system pain, shared something very poignant. "Some people have actually said to me 'At least your condition is not life-threatening'—as if that's supposed to make me feel better. Sometimes I wish this *was* terminal, so there would be an end to my pain."

It may seem that we are asking a lot of you to educate yourself and others at the same time. But suppressing your feelings and emotions can hold back your recovery. Pace yourself, but find at least one person who can give you the compassion and help you need. It's crucial to your recovery to receive as much emotional support as possible.

WORKING THINGS OUT AT WORK

Lucy—the fashion magazine editor who suffers from pelvic floor dysfunction—says, "I have to leave work all the time for medical appointments, and I can't tell them why. I am stressed about 95 percent of the time because of how this problem affects my work. I hate that I have to keep this part of my life a secret, because I am normally a very open person, and I don't like secrets. But I don't feel comfortable sharing this with anyone at work, or with anyone other than my sister."

If figuring out how much to share is tough with loved ones, how much harder is it to figure out for the people you work with? You actually have three problems:

- establishing your need for medical appointments and arranging for other accommodations with your employer;

- coming to some kind of arrangement with coworkers who are affected by your absences; and

- maintaining closeness with workmates who are also friends.

Once again, the key to figuring out what to do is to start with yourself and your own feelings. How much do you want to share? There are always ways to convey that you have medical needs without going into detail. Your doctor can write a letter to your employer about your pain condition that doesn't divulge the exact details of your medical diagnoses. Here's one way you might present your situation:

I need to let you know that I'm dealing with some medical problems. I don't want to go into details, but it's not cancer or anything life-threatening. It's not contagious; and we are looking forward to a full recovery, though I don't yet have a timeline for you. It does sometimes involve severe pain, and I may need some medical procedures, but I'm sure I can work everything out and get all my work done. I'd rather keep all of this private, but I'm happy to bring you a doctor's letter if you need it for your records.

Depending on your condition, you might be able to give alternate reasons for the accommodations you need. For instance, if your condition causes pain with prolonged sitting, you can tell your boss or coworkers that you have hip or low-back pain instead. If you need to sit on a specially designed pillow, you can refer to orthopedic or muscle pain without going into details.

If you need specific accommodations—such as time off—and you can manage that financially and without jeopardizing your job, you may have to ask your employer or a human resources executive to arrange it for you. Here are some suggestions for how you might proceed:

- Figure out ahead of time what you are going to say, and decide exactly how much time you need off.

- Decide whether you want total disability or part-time disability (i.e., time in which you're completely away from work, or just reduced hours).

- Ask your doctor to write a letter recommending time off and giving a diagnosis that doesn't have to be specific, such as hip pain, low-back pain, or pelvic pain.

Work can be an enjoyable and ego-gratifying part of your life. So if you can remain at your job with adjustments and adaptations, that might be a satisfying choice. Although sometimes nothing helps you forget about your pain, you might find that your work distracts you and gives you a sense of purpose.

However, when pelvic pain severely restricts your ability to work, taking some time off might help you heal. In Deborah's experience, patients who take three to six months of temporary disability leave are able to pursue medical treatments and consultations in a way that wouldn't have been possible with full-time work. If this is your decision, you might be able to concentrate on physical therapy, a home exercise program, and other healing activities that will allow your recovery to happen more quickly. This is not a vacation, but time that you deserve to fully investigate your condition and to use your energy to heal. Pain limits and saps energy, so you need to save your resources for your recovery.

Living with intense pain is exhausting, and time off from a stressful or tiring job will help you get better sleep and reduce your stress. Many studies on sleep show that lack of sleep has a deleterious effect on many organs that are involved in pain conditions. Several muscles in the pelvic floor are only able to rest during sleep, because they are needed constantly during daily activities. The central nervous system and the pelvic nerves also need time off from firing. And of course, sleep benefits the immune system and chronic inflammation. So if all you accomplish during your disability leave is getting adequate sleep, you have already taken an enormous step on your healing journey.

When it comes to deciding what to tell your coworkers, you'll again be balancing the possible advantages of openness with your own wish for privacy. Of course, your medical condition is nobody's business. But if you're going to be absent for doctor's appointments or on days that the pain is especially bad—or if you need other kinds of accommodations from coworkers, you might want to give them some explanation, if only to make your own life easier.

If your relationships at work have already suffered due to your absences, don't worry. You can repair them over time as you recover. Focus on getting well, and don't expect yourself to solve every problem at once. After you're feeling better, you'll have more physical and emotional energy to restore and repair relationships.

BEING HONEST WITH YOURSELF

Some women feel that the only way they can save face and not completely fall apart is to repress many of their negative emotions. If you are denying or suppressing any of your difficult or painful feelings, we are here to tell you—gently—that you may be making a mistake. Repressing, denying, or suppressing your feelings is not only ineffective, but it can also actually perpetuate your physical pain.

Emotions have not caused your condition, but keeping your feelings to yourself can cause you so much distress and tension that your pain may intensify as you tense up with the effort of holding everything in. Release your feelings through a pain journal, yoga, meditation, spiritual or religious contemplation, time with a friend or a therapist, or in any way that works for you—but do find some way to let yourself know and accept what you're really feeling, even if you don't want to share your feelings with anyone you know.

WORKING IT OUT WITH A PARTNER

As we saw in the previous chapter, sexual pain can create rifts in an intimate relationship, over and above any specific sexual difficulties.

For example, Blair, a teacher in her early fifties, has a very supportive and loving husband but told us that her sexual pain had deeply affected her feelings about herself. "I felt that I had to be 'on' with my husband, sexually and emotionally, and I couldn't do it. I had a lot of guilt about that. I turned off at home after a long day of work, and that was a tremendous source of frustration to my husband. Sometimes I need to be solitary after a day of pain. The pain changed our habits of relating to each other."

How do you maintain an intimate relationship under such difficult conditions? Here are a few suggestions.

Maintain open and honest communication.

The most important part of dealing with sexual pain is communication. It is vital to let your partner know how you are feeling about all the issues and emotions that affect you—especially your sexual identity, damaged sense of self, anxiety, depression, sexual activity, and difficulties coping with the activities of daily living.

After all, your sexual pain affects virtually every aspect of your life, including your ability to sit, which clothes you can wear, how you take care of household chores, how you fulfill your childcare responsibilities, and how you handle your job. Your partner needs to know how these things affect you. You should not assume he or she knows what you are feeling; instead, you need to share your feelings explicitly.

Also, because your pain might vary from day to day or even hour to hour, you might find it useful to rely on pain scoring, using a scale of 1 to 10. Beth, the freelance writer in her late forties, says that her husband appreciates knowing what her pain level is on a daily basis, so that when he walks through the door, he doesn't "have to read her mind" or guess how she is feeling and what help she may need.

Let them help.

There are many areas of your life where you now require assistance, such as cooking, taking care of the house, and taking care of your children. You are not weak if you ask for help! You have a medical condition that at times may make it difficult for you to attend to activities that you normally do. It's very important that you share all your concerns and needs with your partner and ask for help.

Beth was at times in such agonizing pain that she could not always maintain the level of energy she was accustomed to. "I am a very independent and determined woman and have a tough time asking people for help. But there were times when my pain was so agonizing that even driving to pick up my children from an afternoon activity became too monumental a task for me to handle. I am very fortunate to have such a wonderful and caring husband who never minimized my pain and knew that I was truly suffering. So there were times when he had to pick up the slack at home and with taking care of the kids."

You might find it helpful to schedule time to sit and talk with your partner and share what each of you needs in the relationship. Please don't ever worry about appearing weak or needy. You are not whining or complaining but are having normal reactions to a debilitating and overwhelming situation.

Educate your partner.

It's important that your partner be as knowledgeable as possible about your condition, both because information is empowering, and because your partner needs to understand what you are experiencing.

Remember they are suffering too.

If your partner sometimes seems to withdraw or shut down, it may be that they too are overwhelmed by dealing with your pain.

Beth is very much aware that her husband is still devastated by everything she went through and is still going through. "Sometimes when I want to talk about my emotional and physical experiences, he just shuts down," she says. "I don't get upset; I get that he has been through hell and back, and sometimes reliving our pain is too much for him."

Beth recalls discussions with her husband when she was in debilitating pain. "He sometimes said to me 'I know what you are going through.' I told him how angry that made me, because there was no way that he could know how horrible my pain was. But I also told him that I couldn't imagine how difficult it was for him to watch me in pain, and he was able to share his feelings of sadness, helplessness, and fear. These moments—when we really talked—are what saved our marriage," she says.

Let each other fall apart—but try to not collapse at the same time!
There are times when allowing yourself to temporarily fall apart is actually therapeutic. You cannot possibly maintain the same level of emotional balance and physical resilience that you did before your pain condition began. You are experiencing loss, even if only temporary, on so many levels—loss of the person you were, loss of your sense of safety in your body, loss of your normal activities and socializing, loss of your ability to easily engage in sex without thinking about it. So you will actually go through a grief process that at times requires that you retreat from the world.

It's important that you let your partner know these are normal responses to the pain and loss you're both experiencing. As we see it, a temporary emotional collapse is like recharging your cell phone battery. Your cell phone won't function without being recharged, and neither will you. Sometimes recharging means taking a break from the world, and sometimes it means you need more physical and emotional comfort. Whatever you need is fine—there is no right or wrong in this situation. However, the key to maintaining your relationship is letting your partner know what you need and educating him or her about normal reactions to an abnormal situation.

Ask for reassurance if you need it—and help your partner learn how to give it.

Although you need empathy, you also may need your partner to be a cheerleader and to give you hope. Blair, who suffers from pelvic floor dysfunction, recalled needing her husband to give her frequent reassurance. "I would sometimes ask my husband five times a day for reassurance that I will get better," she says. "I would also say how sorry I was for being such a nudge, but I needed him telling me that to keep me going."

Dave is the boyfriend of Lucy, who suffers from pelvic floor dysfunction. He says, "One of the hardest parts of this situation is balancing intimacy while trying not to pressure Lucy into something she is not comfortable with. We need to talk about this a lot so we don't become alienated from each other." Dave also shared his frustration about not being able to fix Lucy's problem. "When I see a problem, I usually want to try to fix it, but with this, I feel powerless," he says. "I try to reassure her every time she is frustrated—with physical therapy or with all the medication she has to take—that she is doing what she needs to do to fix this." This is an example of the frustration men often feel as a result of their "fix-it" mentality—and this also shows how important the "cheerleader" role is in this situation.

Have compassion—for both of you.

When you experience sexual pain, you and your partner have entered into a journey for which you are totally unprepared. Your relationship will definitely be affected. However, your pain condition does not have to define you or your relationship. You will have to work hard at keeping your relationship vibrant, but with sensitivity, compassion, understanding, communication, and empathy, your partner and you can successfully navigate the challenges you face.

A PARTNER SPEAKS

Blair's husband, Tom, has been supportive of his wife throughout her ordeal, but he agrees that their relationship has been shaken by what she went through. He also continues to struggle with the problems it presents.

"I find it the hardest to provide emotional support when I experience physical or emotional stress of my own," he admits. "I sometimes get very frustrated when Blair's medical condition becomes the center of our life.

"I never feel any guilt about her condition; I just feel sad for her. Her ailment is so mysterious. I usually don't feel a lot of anger about her condition—it's more frustration. I also don't feel responsible for Blair's condition; I just feel concerned.

"I don't ever feel that I have sexual difficulties as a result of Blair's sexual pain, but I do feel some apprehension and guilt when I do pursue any form of sex. I don't worry about touching her in the wrong places, because she tells me where it's okay to touch and where it's not."

How does Tom cope with this incredibly stressful situation? "I go to the gym, focus on my well-being, watch sports, read newspapers, attend concerts, and go to the beach. I cannot focus all my attention on our problem—that would detract from our relationship and make me very emotionally unhealthy."

Tom spoke about the dilemma of burdening Blair with his feelings. "I worry about burdening her with my emotional concerns and feelings. We discuss my feelings and concerns at certain times when it has been warranted. But it's not useful or constructive to be stuck in the same discussion over and over again.

"It seems that when one obstacle is solved, another arises. That can make me feel very hopeless at times. But luckily my wife is persistent and resilient. She keeps the hope alive. I do

➤

> worry that we will never be able to have intercourse normally again. That scares me. And when I get really hopeless, I need to detach, knowing her resiliency makes this a temporary event."
>
> When we asked Tom what advice he would give to partners of women suffering from sexual pain, he said, "Be patient, compassionate, understanding—and listen. And also, don't forget to take care of yourself. Treat yourself to things you enjoy. Acknowledge that the whole family gets affected."

TALKING TO YOUR CHILDREN

Even young children notice when a parent isn't feeling well, so your children are bound to have some feelings about your condition. And when children know there's a problem and no one admits it, they feel even more anxious. If you don't tell them, your "mysterious" condition may become so frightening that it may cause excessive anxiety and depression. Keeping secrets from children is never a good idea—their thoughts take on a life of their own and make your situation even harder for them to cope with. When they see you not acting like yourself and perhaps not taking care of them as you usually do, they might also worry that you have cancer or some other life-threatening condition.

We strongly recommend telling your children what's going on, in a way that's appropriate to their ages. Just speak simply and honestly, and let your children know how they will be affected. You might also let them know that any feelings they have about your condition are okay, and that they should feel comfortable asking you any questions or sharing any concerns. Of course, tell them that you're getting help for your condition, and that you're confident you will improve.

Here are some practical suggestions for speaking with your children:

• Describe your condition in simple terms.

• Emphasize that the pain is not their fault or your fault, and that they can't catch what you have.

• Assure them that your life is not in danger, and that you're working with a doctor to help you feel better.

• Let your children know that pain can be unpredictable. Tell them that sometimes Mommy may be fine, but other times she might not be able to participate in certain activities.

• Reassure them that your situation is only temporary, and that you will get better.

• Tell them about any scheduling changes you have to make while you seek care. But let them know there will always be someone who loves them to care for them.

• Let your children know that no feelings are wrong or bad, and that anything they feel is fine with you. Tell them that you get sad and angry at times, and that they might have the same feelings.

• Tell your children how hopeful you feel about your ability to get better.

WHEN THE PAIN IS GONE

We've talked about what you can do to heal your relationships while you are struggling with sexual pain, and our advice is very similar for the period after you have begun to recover—when the pain is receding but the painful memories are still present.

You may feel at this point as though you have an enormous amount of repair work to do: with your romantic relationship, among family and friends, at work, perhaps even with your children. It will take you and every-body else some time to get used to the fact that you now can take good health and pain-free days for granted, that you can move on to the things you used to do before you got sick.

Our best advice is to take it slow, to keep being honest with yourself about how you feel, and to treat yourself and everyone else with compassion. Most likely, no one handled your illness perfectly, including you. Probably there are some hurt feelings, some frustrations, and some unfinished business in more than one relationship—whether it's you wishing you had handled things differently, or the other person wishing they had risen to the occasion better, or perhaps both of you still harboring resentment or frustration that may have more to do with the stress that surrounds a severe illness than with anything else.

Even if ostensibly everything is fine, it will probably take time for you to get used to socializing again, to having sex, to being able to function as you used to—or almost as you used to—at home and work. The healing journey is a long one, often with twists and turns, but if you are committed to your own health and the health of your relationships, you will re-create the joy-ous, fulfilling life that you deserve.

16

MOVING FORWARD

I can't give up hope. I don't believe that I was ever meant to suffer like this forever, and that there has to be an end to my agony. I don't think I will ever be pain-free, but I have to believe that some treatment is out there to alleviate some of my pain and help me lead a more normal life.

—SANDRA, BIOMEDICAL TECHNICIAN, AGE THIRTY-THREE

Living with pain can help you take things you previously took for granted and perceive them differently. I continue to struggle with intense and frequent pain, and at the moment, I'm not certain what my prospects are, medically. But I still have hope. And meanwhile, the daily moments of my life mean the world to me. For example, putting my son to bed sometimes takes on a mystical quality. When we read books together and he tells me how much he loves me, my heart soars. And even though my life is very far from perfect, I realize how lucky I am to have these encounters with my child.

—MARY, A TEACHER IN HER FORTIES

OW DO YOU recover from the trauma of sexual pain—a physical and emotional ordeal that affected every area of your life, and that, even now, may not be completely over? How do you stop worrying that the pain might someday recur, or start viewing your body and your sexuality as sources of pleasure rather than torment? How do you claim an identity that isn't primarily about your pain, or return to a set of relationships with people who might have no idea of what you have been through and certainly have never been through anything similar themselves?

These are not easy questions for the survivor of any trauma. Soldiers who have seen combat, families who have lived through natural disasters, individuals who have suddenly or violently lost loved ones or who have themselves been victims of an attack—you, the sexual-pain survivor, now join their ranks, even as you retain your own unique experience and your own special problems.

As with other types of trauma, there are no easy answers, and there is no single response. Perhaps you'll enjoy a complete physical recovery from sexual pain and still bear some of the scars from your experience—perhaps from pain and from medical mistreatment. Perhaps you'll continue to suffer from some form of chronic pain in various degrees of intensity. Perhaps you'll alternate between days of no pain and unpredictable flare-ups. Or perhaps you will one day find yourself completely healed, physically and emotionally, no longer able to quite remember the ordeal that now seems to dominate your life.

As with any serious or chronic illness, no one—neither you nor your physician—can easily predict the outcome of your condition. But we can say with certainty that there are many possibilities for treatment, and that new, more effective approaches to sexual pain are being discovered all the time. However—particularly if your sexual pain has neurological or orthopedic roots—you may be faced with some ongoing level of pain.

The two of us now spend our professional lives working with women who struggle with sexual and other types of chronic pain, and Nancy faces her own ongoing battle with pelvic pain. From the depths of our own experience, we want to offer you two potential sources of hope. One is the very real possibility that you will find a way to completely recover from your emotional and physical trauma, and that you'll go on to a pain-free life. The other is that even if you continue to experience some physical pain and emotional challenges, you can still lead a productive, meaningful, and satisfying life, filled with relationships, activities, and experiences that you treasure.

FINDING PERSPECTIVE

How do you arrive at that perspective, able to cherish elements of your life even while struggling with pain? Each of us must find her own answer. But the two of us have found strength through our own personal struggles by focusing on achieving meaning through intimate relationships, work that has a positive effect on others, spiritual satisfaction, and a true connection with the people in our lives.

Happiness is not defined by how much leisure time we are able to fit into our stressful lives, or by the most expensive car we can afford to buy. Happiness is defined by the small but precious moments that we sometimes take for granted. When your colleague or employee says, "Thank you for your guidance"; when your partner tells you, "I am here for you no matter what"; when your friend says, "I would do anything for you; just tell me what it is"; or when your child announces, "My teacher told me I said the smartest thing in class today!"—those are the moments that make your life worth living, even in the face of pain.

If you could feel this way every day in the face of chronic pain, you would fit our definition of a saint or a superhuman—and we've never met a woman who was either. But if you can feel this way at least *some* of the time, you can find a way to weave your loss, grief, and trauma into a new tapestry that allows you to value and even enjoy the meaning in your life.

POSSIBLE RESPONSES TO
THE TRAUMA OF SEXUAL PAIN

If you're feeling one or more of the following, you're not alone:

- alienation from your own body, especially from your sexual organs and sexual feelings;

- anxiety, distrust, anger, or contempt for the medical system and for physicians;

- vulnerability and an ongoing awareness that you can't take your health or safety for granted;

- lowered libido, desire, and sexual responsiveness; and/or

- grief for your lost ability to take your sexual well-being for granted, or to assume that you're "entitled" to a life without pain.

IF YOU HAVE RECOVERED FROM SEXUAL PAIN

If you're able to live each day without being consumed by pain and are able to enjoy sexual intimacy once again, you have a lot to be grateful for. However, you might still retain some form of permanent trauma, or at least feel marked by the experience. Cancer survivors often speak of their illness as a defining event: Forever after, their lives are divided into "life before" and "life after" cancer. You may experience something similar with sexual pain—perhaps for some months after the experience, perhaps for longer.

For example, Miriam is one of our patients who was completely cured of her vestibulodynia. But she emerged from her ordeal feeling "amputated." She felt as though her sexuality and her anatomy had become medicalized— that she had developed a public persona that could speak freely about her body and her sex life, but that her true, intimate, vulnerable, sensual self was in hiding, far from the doctors and their instruments. Having recovered from her physical pain, Miriam then faced another challenge: to reconnect with "the person hiding in the corner" and reclaim her sexual self.

As you recuperate from the ordeal you've endured, we encourage you to accept your feelings, whatever they might be. Don't let anyone tell you that you are being oversensitive, that you should just put these thoughts out of your mind, or that you need to "just move on and get over it." You are entitled to all of your feelings, and repressing them would be unhealthy.

Having said that, you should also know that your feelings don't have to control your life. You have some choices about how to handle them. Their intensity should ease as you move along in the recovery process, so if you feel stuck, overwhelmed, or lost, we urge you to get help—ideally from a therapist trained in chronic pain and trauma issues, or possibly from a religious or spiritual leader or a support group.

Another aspect of recovery may well include regaining at least some measure of comfort with, if not confidence in, the medical system. You will need healthcare practitioners the rest of your life for conditions that are totally unrelated to your sexual pain. Even if you have had negative experiences with physicians, please remember that there are many good doctors out there. However, you can view your problematic experiences with physicians as a learning experience—you are now more educated about the medical system and will be able to make better choices when it comes to ascertaining the kind of doctors you want in your life.

Perhaps the most important element in your ultimate emotional recovery is your own commitment to finding meaning in your experience. Although you have gone through unspeakable and undeserved trauma that you did not choose, you do have a choice about what to do with all that you have learned, intellectually and emotionally, from the experience. Although you were powerless over what happened to you, paradoxically, your experience can empower you. Perhaps you'll be more sensitive to other people's emotions and will therefore become a better friend. Maybe you can advocate for someone who is totally lost in the medical system. Perhaps your ordeal will somehow transform your relationship with your work, your loved ones, or yourself.

The worst thing that could result from your sexual pain is to become embittered and further defeated by your pain. Of course, you have a right to be angry and feel a sense of loss. But we urge you not to let negativity overtake you and define your entire relationship to the world.

RECLAIMING YOUR SEXUAL SELF

You need to give yourself time to regain your sense of sexuality—but you can actively help in the process. Here are some more suggestions for helping yourself feel sexual again:

- List all your wonderful qualities that make you a sexual and attractive woman.

- Ask your partner or your loved ones to tell you three sexy and attractive things about you.

- Take a class that opens you sexually, such as Zumba, bellydancing, or tango.

- Create affirmations to remind you that your sexuality does not stem from your vulva or vagina but from your inner sense of self.

- Dress up for a date with your partner and have a romantic evening.

CONTRACEPTION

Once you have experienced sexual pain, you may worry that a pregnancy may exacerbate your symptoms or renew symptoms that have completely disappeared. This worry of course may decrease your libido and sexual enjoyment. To avoid this, use a good contraceptive method. Here are some pointers about each:

HORMONAL CONTRACEPTION

This easily available choice includes oral pills, external patches, injectables, implants, or vaginal rings. We have advised many women to stop or sometimes to start hormonal contraception as part of their treatment of different conditions, and many have been able to return to this method once they are healed. Others fear doing this and would rather use another method. Work with your physician to figure out the choices that are right for you.

CONDOMS

These remain your best method, since they put no long-lasting chemicals into your body and are only temporarily in contact with your tissues. Of course, if you are dating or not in a mutually monogamous relationship, you must use them to protect yourself from sexually transmitted infections. If you or your committed partner have tried several types to give them a full chance and still dislike them, you have some other options.

THE MIRENA IUD

This offers you contraception that will last for a few years. Gaining rapidly in popularity, it has the added benefit of markedly

➤

reducing menstrual flow and, for many women, cramps. That's a real benefit: fewer pads and tampons to irritate you, and less need for pain medications around your menses.

THE DIAPHRAGM

This is not a good choice for most of our patients, unfortunately. It requires spermicide, which can irritate the genitals; it must stay in for several hours, which can also cause irritation; and it puts pressure on the bladder and pelvic floor muscles. But if you have been using it without trouble, and you like it, by all means, continue.

THE CERVICAL CAP

This is available again in the United States and may be more comfortable than the diaphragm, since it is smaller and needs less spermicide. However, it is still a vaginal device and it may irritate the vaginal canal, but do try it if you are interested.

THE FEMALE CONDOM

Though it never gained popularity due to its awkwardness, newer, better versions are in the pipeline, so be on the lookout. It might be helpful for you in the future.

PERMANENT STERILIZATION

This is an option for women who don't ever want to get pregnant, or conceive again. But we perform fewer of these procedures than before, because Mirena is now so popular and provides easy long-term contraception.

IF YOU ARE STILL COPING WITH SEXUAL PAIN

If you're still recovering from sexual pain, you may face many of the same emotional challenges as women who have already recovered—along with a special set of difficulties, such as the following:

- unpredictable pain flare-ups;

- keeping up with medical appointments, treatments, and self-education;

- ongoing effects of pain on your work life;

- depression and hopelessness about your life ever getting better;

- frequent thoughts of suicide;

- ongoing stress in your relationships;

- dealing with the idea of having to continue to live with a certain degree of pain;

- trouble getting pleasure and meaning in life; and/or

- living and coping as a "complicated patient."

Unpredictable Flare-Ups

One of the hardest parts of living with pain is its unpredictability. It's bad enough having to avoid activities that you know might set off your pain, such as a long car drive, a long work session, or going to a movie. But to experience unprovoked pain with no idea what set it off is extremely demoralizing, frustrating, and stressful.

So how do you keep pain from dictating every aspect of your life? The worst outcome would be for you to let pain define who you are and how you live. Of course, pain does affect you, and you will have to accommodate its presence in your life. But there are ways to minimize your modifications and continue to engage in activities you enjoy.

We'll be honest with you: When you're having a high-level pain day, there is little you can do but get through the day. We will not ask you to find ways to be happy or even content. Some days you just have to take it hour by hour—some days, even that is too much to ask.

But there are days when your pain is more moderate, when going out to dinner and a movie may indeed be possible. Trite as it sounds, you just need to take life one day at a time. When you are having good days, take advantage of them and do things you love to do. Go ahead and make some plans for the future—such as dinner out with friends or a movie with your kids. Accept that you may need to cancel some plans, and give yourself permission to stay home and pamper yourself if you need to. Be aware that sometimes—even when you're having a very painful day—one of the best things you can do is to distract yourself. Only you can judge how to balance these two possibilities. The important thing is that you not give up on enjoying those things you can enjoy. That would be a true defeat.

We know that we're asking you to show a tremendous amount of courage, determination, and strength. But always giving in to your pain allows that pain to define you, to create an "illness identity," where the illness becomes you. You stop being a woman who loves to walk in the woods, who does interesting work, who has strong opinions about current events or politics or movies or relationships, and who often struggles with pain, and become instead "someone with sexual pain." Resisting that self-definition is challenging and may sometimes be more than you can handle. But don't ever start to believe that you and your illness are one and the same.

Keeping Up with Medical Appointments, Treatments, and Self-Education

Obviously, you need to keep your appointments and undergo treatments—but no one is saying you have to like them. What can make things easier is finding healthcare practitioners who are compassionate and understanding. As we discussed in Chapter 3, even when you find a competent physician, you may not feel personally attached to him or her. However, it may be easier to find a physical therapist you like personally as well as professionally, and that should make one portion of your healthcare far easier to manage,

nal stenosis, which caused horrendous pain down her sciatic nerve. Her
var pain also became much worse.

"At this point, my emotional state was, to say the least, not good," Beth
ys. "I had finally felt that I was beginning to recover, and now I was back
a life of pain, back in my own little corner of hell."

Despite her trepidation, Beth underwent microsurgery on her back.
The first few weeks of recovery was hell. My nerve pain was so bad," Beth
ecalls. "Just making it through every second of every day was a monumental feat."

At about four months after the operation, after intense physical therapy,
Beth felt about 90 percent better. At last, she thought, she had turned the
corner.

"I finally felt like I was getting my life back," she says. "I was working
out at the gym doing the elliptical and upper- and lower-body weights, and I
was beginning to feel like the person I was five years ago. My goal is still to
return to long-distance bike riding and tennis, which I miss terribly. Biking
for me was therapeutic, an escape from the emotional pain in my life. My
two-hour bike rides on an early Sunday morning were so liberating. That
was one of the things I missed most when I was sick."

But Beth's ordeal was not yet over. She soon noticed some vulvar burning and itching near the rectal area. She had developed another set of complications that required yet another surgery. "Now I had to disrupt my life
once again, and return to crutches, and stop my exercise routine once again,
and go back to rehabilitative physical therapy," she says.

Like many complicated patients, Beth needed validation for her feelings of anger, depression, and resentment—while also wanting hope that
she would once again be better. "Although the physical pain was much less
during my recuperation, my emotional state was severely affected. I didn't
want to see people and didn't even want to be around my family. I was so
resentful about everything that I just wanted to be left alone.

"I also felt a tremendous amount of guilt about not being able to
take care of my children, once again. In this case, practice does not make

if not actually enjoyable. Many women we know become so emotionally
connected to their physical therapist that they don't want to reduce the frequency of appointments, even when they're able to do so. It's great when
your physical therapist can become part of your emotional support system.

If you hate or dread or even simply dislike any portion of your medical
treatment, of course those feelings are valid. It may be helpful to remind
yourself that even though you have a right to resent this part of your life, you
must also embrace it, because it is part of helping yourself get better. Try to
treat yourself after each appointment with something pleasurable, like visiting your favorite café, getting ice cream, or getting a manicure. You need to
pamper yourself as much as possible.

It is important that you keep up with the research and advancements in
the field of chronic sexual pain. At your medical visits, ask your doctor about
any new information, and share what you may have read with him or her.
The best and easiest way to stay abreast of the improvements in treatment
is to become a member of the National Vulvodynia Association (NVA). The
NVA's multifaceted mission includes educating and providing a support network for members, as well as advocating and supporting research and the
education of the medical community and general public. We urge you to
join. See the Resources section for contact information.

If You Are a Complicated Patient

Most sexual-pain patients recover substantially and can live their lives with
no pain or very limited pain. But what if you're in that small percentage of
women who have more complicated situations, with pain that is extremely
difficult to treat? What if you have endured multiple procedures, taken hundreds of medications, and seen numerous specialists—and have achieved
some pain relief at times, but are seemingly locked into a nightmarish pattern of taking two steps forward and then two steps back?

We still believe there is significant hope for you, because there is so
much scientific research being conducted. We want to tell you that you are in
no way destined to live a life riddled with debilitating pain. But sometimes,

honestly, we feel at a loss. Even while we want to support your sense of hope and optimism, we're well aware that you have endured and continue to endure more pain than anyone should in a lifetime.

In order to protect yourself from more disappointment and failed procedures, you are allowed sometimes to almost completely give up hope. You can say to yourself, "There is nothing out there that will help me, and I will probably live in horrible pain for the rest of my life." You might even say to yourself that at some point, you might have to make a choice: Either figure out a way to live with this pain or actually end your life. Sometimes your physical and emotional resources are so drained, and you have lived through so much disappointment—how could you feel or think any differently?

So we give you permission to give up hope, to consider suicide, and to view every treatment as a potential failure. This may sound nontherapeutic or even possibly unethical. But we are going to tell you that giving yourself permission to think in this way is probably the most therapeutic and effective tactic you can take.

First, you need to voice these feelings to someone who cares about you and whom you can trust. Keeping these feelings to yourself is destructive.

Second, we're pleading with you that, in the midst of this hopelessness and despair, you continue to pursue treatments, because you never know when there is that one treatment that might be able to lessen the severity of your pain. We know you don't really want to give up. Your hopelessness is only a way of saying that you're so emotionally depleted that expressing or actually feeling hope is too difficult or scary.

You can allow yourself to sink into a pit of despair, but at the same time, try to say to yourself, "I do want to live, and I have so much to live for." Allow the people in your life who love and cherish you to give you support and to push you to pursue and endure that next treatment.

This may sound contradictory, but it actually isn't. We know you don't want to end your life or give up. But there are times when it is too much of us to ask you to maintain that unfailing hope. We feel confident that your hopelessness will be a temporary state.

Still, to endure that next treatment, medication, you sometimes must enter a state of self-protection even no expectations. At the same time, you must sea heart and say, "Until there is no hope, there is hope." U yourself, "My life is truly not worth living, and there is that I treasure," then you have to follow that one small p and keep on living your life.

Yes, you have suffered more than anyone should be as have experienced more physical and emotional setbacks tha have in their lifetime. But your heart will not let you stop tryi to others who can understand your pain, and we implore you some basic level, that your search will result in a lessening of y and emotional pain. We are asking you to use superhuman s somewhere inside of you, we believe you have the ability to hang maintain the belief that your life is worth living.

A COMPLICATED PATIENT: BETH'S STORY

Beth is a freelance writer in her late forties. Her long, involved hi sexual pain exemplifies the problems faced by the complicated patie

Initially, Beth was struggling with a tear in her hip labrum. Afte surgery, the pain lessened markedly. Beth's state of mind improved as though she was also worried about the extent to which she would rec Any pain that she experienced caused tremendous anxiety, as she asked self whether it was the beginning of a downward spiral that would u mately condemn her to a lifetime of intense pain.

But her improvement continued. "I told both Dr. Coady and my orth pedic surgeon that they saved my life. If I didn't have the surgery, I don' know if I would have lived, because I couldn't tolerate living in such agonizing pain. I told them both they gave me my life back."

Then, while recovering, Beth suffered a back injury that was set off by how her surgery had changed her body mechanics. She was diagnosed with perfect. The more that was thrown on my plate, the harder it was to bounce back. No matter how hard I tried to be positive during my recuperation, I still felt intense resentment and anger that I had to go through this once again.

"I was also scared, because I didn't know how long it would take for me to get past this anger. I knew in the long run I was going to be okay, but I was so, so angry I had to be in this place again and go through the whole physical therapy routine again.

"One of my kids was so angry that I had to have another surgery and that she had to see me on crutches that she basically left the house for the week and found different places to stay. I let her know her feelings were okay and gave her permission to do whatever she needed to do. I think that helped her a great deal."

Like many complicated patients, Beth spent weeks thinking about suicide. To cope, she created a visual image of her children going off on the bus without her kissing them goodbye. That image kept her from actually coming up with a plan. We think that patients like Beth are afraid to be too hopeful, because every time they work with such determination and perseverance to get better, they then seem to have another medical setback. We have to treat complicated patients delicately—never minimizing their feelings but also trying to help them overcome the trauma they have gone through. We need to help them see that although they have been through so much, this is not their plight in life.

It is hard for a woman like Beth—who considered herself to be such a vibrant and healthy person—to be continuously thrown into the role of the infirm. It will be a huge task for Beth to regain her healthy and active persona. But she's doing the right things.

"I know talking to my therapist is the best way to get back on track and to give myself time," Beth says. "I know I had every right to have all these feelings, and that I have to be patient with myself and ask everyone else to be patient with me. I know that I will have to work very hard to regain my sense of emotional and physical health—and at times, I won't want to work that hard. . . . In the long run—because I am a fighter and very resilient—I will be fine. But returning to my former self will be a monumental task."

Beth's story is not typical. Most of you reading this book will never face the setbacks and complications she has endured—but some of you will. For all of you—those who enjoy a complete recovery, those who enjoy a partial recovery, and those few who are in Beth's situation—we hope you'll find inspiration in Beth's commitment to never giving up, to always seeking a better solution, and to continually finding meaning and joy, even in the face of pain.

Ongoing Effects of Pain on Your Work Life

In Chapter 15, there are many specific suggestions for handling work issues. Here we just want to remind you of your right to maintain your privacy at whatever level you choose, and of your right to continue asking for accommodations for as long as you need them. Sometimes when a condition has gone on for a while, either you or your coworkers may start to feel, "Enough already! This should be over." If anyone begins to feel that way and the pain still doesn't stop, you end up in an impossible situation: You can't make the pain go away, and you can't stop needing the accommodations.

What can make the situation somewhat better is your own complete clarity that you have not done anything wrong, you have not chosen this pain, you are not malingering or using your illness to get special attention, and you have every right to continue working with whatever accommodations you need. In fact, you have a basic human right to sexual and reproductive health, as even the World Health Organization stated in their 2003 updated human rights statement: Reproductive rights rest on the recognition of the basic right of all couples and individuals to decide freely and responsibly the number, spacing, and timing of their children and to have the information and means to do so, and the right to attain the highest standard of sexual and reproductive health. They also include the right of all to make decisions concerning reproduction free of discrimination, coercion, and violence. (www.who.int /reproductivehealth/en)

We know it can be challenging at times, but if you take this attitude, other people are far more likely to fall in with it. Likewise, if you feel uncertain, or if you open yourself to criticism, you make it easier for other people to question you. Try to be clear, committed, and nondefensive about what you need, and you will give yourself the best possible shot at making things go the way you want them to.

Learning to Live with a Certain Degree of Pain

It is not acceptable to live with agonizing pain. And for any degree of pain, you're entitled to all your emotions—including anger, depression, frustration, sadness, and at times, hopelessness. But even though pain will never be your friend, you can find a way to adapt to a certain level. You should never stop actively searching for increasing medical relief—that needs to always be your goal. Remarkably, your body and psyche are so adaptable, that at times, you may not even notice your pain, even though it persists.

Once again, we're asking you to deal with a contradictory situation: to accept your pain and adapt to it, even as you continue working with your doctors to reduce it. That is your challenge—but it is absolutely a challenge that can be met.

Finding Ways to Enjoy Life

The secret of getting pleasure and meaning from your life is easy to state though hard to practice: Don't view anything in your life as trivial.

Going out to lunch with a friend, listening to music, sitting by the ocean, playing a game with your child—any of these experiences, even if you are in pain, can be deeply meaningful and even miraculous.

You can also find pleasure and meaning in work and community. You can find extraordinary meaning in self-expression, communal expression, serving others, or promoting a higher ideal if you find your work satisfying; if you're engaged in volunteer activities; if you take part in a political, environmental, or religious community; or if you have other ways of making your voice heard in the world.

Never minimize the importance of the close relationships in your life and how valuable they are. A friend who offers to cook you a meal or a partner who takes you out for a special dinner are parts of your life you should treasure. If you can learn to view all the good parts of your life with gratitude, then even living with pain cannot rob you of the joy in your life.

FEAR OF PREGNANCY

Whether you are still challenged by sexual pain or have recovered from it, you are likely to be fearful about pregnancy and childbirth—worrying that it will make you worse or set you back into pain again.

But the fact is that there is absolutely no medical evidence that pregnancy and childbirth will make your sexual pain worse. In fact, observations show the opposite—that there can be improvement after pregnancy, whether you deliver vaginally or by C-section.

Pregnancy is an anti-inflammatory state and may calm down tissue and nerve inflammation. The increase in blood vessels and thus oxygenation in the pelvis is also helpful for healing. Higher estrogen and other hormone levels are good for the genital skin, mucous membranes, and connective tissues. Muscles, ligaments, and connective tissues relax and lengthen in pregnancy, benefiting pelvic floor balance and loosening nerve restrictions. Endometriosis and other pelvic organ disorders also improve in pregnancy.

So if you want to become a mother, do not let your sexual-pain condition stop your plans. If you worry that you cannot

›

> conceive because you cannot have intercourse, your doctor can provide you with instructions and syringes for home self-insemination, or he or she can perform in-office cervical or intrauterine insemination. Be sure to ask for this help if you need it.

Maintaining Hope

It might seem as though you need to be made out of iron to do all the things that we are asking you to do. And perhaps maintaining hope is the most difficult task of all. However, it is essential that you never totally give up hope.

One thing is certain: It's almost impossible to maintain hope alone. Please find people in your life—professionals and nonprofessionals—who can help give you the strength you need. Moving into the future, with or without pain, is always possible.

Here are some other ways to maintain hope:

- Talk to your doctor about all the research that is being done in the area of sexual pain.

- Visualize the treatments that are not available yet but that may be on the market soon.

- Keep a pain journal. Tracking your pain reminds you that it is changing, that your flare-ups and most intense pain always end, and that you might even be making progress.

- Establish goals for yourself: a new hobby, a book group, some volunteer work, or even a new level of pampering—such as getting a massage on a weekly basis. Goals keep you focused on the future, which may be pain-free, instead of on the painful present.

- Find activities that give your life meaning. You may be grieving the loss of sexual activity, exercise routines, or other physical pursuits, but engaging in activities that take you outside of yourself (like volunteer work, your career, and going out with friends) will give the pain a smaller relative share of your life.

- Give yourself things to look forward to—for example, a trip, a class, a party, or a project. You can plan something extravagant if you want, but even small-scale anticipations can be exciting.

ONE MOMENT AT A TIME

Now that you have the information you need to move forward with your healing journey, what's next? Both the bad news and the good news is that your life will continue to unfold one moment at a time—sometimes shadowed by pain, sometimes lit by joy . . . and sometimes both. Finding hope when you're facing day after day of severe, unremitting pain is a monumental challenge, but you can look forward to relief: medically, psychologically, and sexually.

If you're in an intimate relationship, keep working to find new bridges to intimacy and connection, both sexual and otherwise. If you're single, maintain your faith that love and an intimate relationship are possible for you, and that the person who sees your true gifts for what they are will not be daunted by a medical problem. If you choose to remain single, your goal should also be regaining your sexuality and relief from pain.

In the end, the best advice we can give you is the advice we ourselves have followed on our own healing journeys and life challenges: Educate yourself to the best of your ability, never give up on finding help, build the strongest support network you can, and find meaning in every moment of your life as it unfolds. This isn't always an easy way to live, but it is extremely rewarding—and in the end, it's all any of us can ever do. As fellow travelers along this road, we wish you all the best on your journey.

Although there is no certainty about what lies ahead, if we manage to keep our hopes in the future alive, we will be able to overcome all sorts of difficulties and go on living.

—THE DALAI LAMA

RESOURCES

RECOMMENDED BOOKS

100 Questions & Answers About Life After Breast Cancer: Sensuality, Sexuality, Intimacy, by Michael R. Krychman, MD, Susan Kellogg Spadt, PhD, CRNP, and Sandra Finestone, PsyD (Jones & Bartlett Publishers, 2010).

Body Drama: Real Girls, Real Bodies, Real Issues, Real Answers, by Nancy Amanda Redd (Gotham, 2007)

Cognitive Behavioral Therapy, Second Edition: Basics and Beyond, by Judith S. Beck, PhD, and Aaron T. Beck, MD (The Guilford Press, 2011)

Ending Female Pain: A Woman's Manual—The Ultimate Self-Help Guide for Women Suffering from Chronic Pelvic and Sexual Pain, by Isa Herrera (Duplex Publishing, 2009)

Healing Pelvic Pain: The Proven Stretching, Strengthening, and Nutrition Program for Relieving Pain, Incontinence, IBS, and Other Symptoms without Surgery, by Amy Stein (McGraw-Hill, 2008)

How to Be Sick: A Buddhist-Inspired Guide for the Chronically Ill and Their Caregivers, by Toni Bernhard (Wisdom Publishers, 2010)

Living Well with Pain and Illness: The Mindful Way to Free Yourself from Suffering, by Vidyamala Burch (Sounds True, 2010)

Living with Chronic Pain: The Complete Health Guide to the Causes and Treatment of Chronic Pain, by Jennifer P. Schneider (Hatherleigh Press, 2004)

Masters and Johnson on Sex and Human Loving, by Robert Kolodny, Virginia E. Johnson, and William H. Masters (Little, Brown, 1988)

Mating in Captivity: Unlocking Erotic Intelligence, by Esther Perel (Harper Paperbacks, 2007)

Muscle Medicine: The Revolutionary Approach to Maintaining, Strengthening, and Repairing Your Muscles and Joints, by Rob DeStefano, Joseph Hooper, and Bryan Kelly (Fireside, 2009)

The Orgasm Answer Guide, by Barry R. Komisaruk, Beverly Whipple, Sara Nasserzadeh, and Carlos Beyer-Flores (The Johns Hopkins University Press, 2009)

The Pain Chronicles: Cures, Myths, Mysteries, Prayers, Diaries, Brain Scans, Healing, and the Science of Suffering, by Melanie Thernstrom (Farrar, Strauss & Giroux, 2010)

Pain Solutions, by A. Lee Dellon (Dellon Institutes for Peripheral Nerve Surgery, 2007); also available at www.dellon.com, where it can be downloaded for free

The Psychophysiology of Sex, by Erick Janssen (Kinsey Institute Series, Indiana University Press, 2007)

Sex and Humor: Selections from the Kinsey Institute, by Catherine Johnson, Betsy Stiratt, and John Henry Jeffries Bancroft (Indiana University Press, 2002)

The V Book: A Doctor's Guide to Complete Vulvovaginal Health, by Elizabeth G. Stewart and Paula Spencer (Bantam, 2002)

HELPFUL WEBSITES

The Anti-Inflammatory Diet
www.drweil.com/drw/u/ART02012/anti-inflammatory-diet

Directory of State Medical and Osteopathic Boards
www.fsmb.org/directory_smb.html

The Female Genital Cutting Education and Networking Project
www.fgmnetwork.org/index.php

Hypnosis
www.ibshypnosis.com/IBSclinicians.html

Pelvic Freedom
www.elisabethoas.com/pelvicfreedom

Qigong
www.nqa.org

Sleep
www.ninds.nih.gov/disorders/brain_basics/understanding_sleep.htm

PSYCHOTHERAPISTS

www.psychologytoday.com (click on "Find a Therapist")

RELEVANT ORGANIZATIONS AND ASSOCIATIONS

American Academy of Dermatology (AAD)
PO Box 4014
Schaumburg, IL 60173
(866) 503-7456
www.aad.org

American Academy of Orthopaedic Surgeons (AAOS)
6300 North River Road
Rosemont, IL 60018
(847) 823-7186
www.aaos.org

American Association of Sex Educators, Counselors, and Therapists (AASECT)
1444 I Street NW, Suite 700
Washington, DC 20005
(202) 449-1099
www.aasect.org

American Chronic Pain Association (ACPA)
PO Box 850
Rocklin, CA 95677
(800) 533-3231
www.theacpa.org

American College of Obstetricians and Gynecologists (ACOG)
PO Box 96920
Washington, DC 20090
(202) 638-5577
www.acog.org

American Physical Therapy Association (APTA), Women's Health Section
1111 North Fairfax Street
Alexandria, VA 22314
(800) 999-2782
www.womenshealthapta.org

American Psychological Association (APA)
750 First Street NE
Washington, DC 20002
(800) 374-2741
www.apa.org

British Society for the Study of Vulval Diseases (BSSVD)
www.bssvd.org

The Dellon Institutes for Peripheral Nerve Surgery
1122 Kenilworth Drive
Towson, MD 21204
(410) 337-5400
www.dellon.com

The Endometriosis Association
8585 N. 76th Place
Milwaukee, WI 53223
(414) 355-2200
www.endometriosisassn.org

Endometriosis Foundation of America (EFA)
872 Fifth Avenue
New York, NY 10065
(212) 988-4160 or (845) 987-4247
www.endofound.org

International Pelvic Pain Society (IPPS)
2 Woodfield Lake
1100 E. Woodfield Road, Suite 20
Schaumburg, IL 60173
(847) 517-8712
www.pelvicpain.org

International Society for Sexual Medicine
www.issm.info

International Society for the Study of Vulvovaginal Disease (ISSVD)
8814 Peppergrass Lane
Waxhaw, NC 28173
(704) 814-9493
www.issvd.org

International Society for the Study of Women's Sexual Health (ISSWSH)
2 Woodfield Lake
1100 E. Woodfield Road, Suite 520
Schaumburg, IL 60123
(847) 517-7225
www.isswsh.org

Interstitial Cystitis Network (Painful Bladder Syndrome)
PO Box 2159
Healdsburg, CA 95448
(707) 538-9442
www.ic-network.com

National Association of Cognitive–Behavioral Therapists (NACBT)
PO Box 2195
Weirton, WV 26062
(800) 853-1135
www.nacbt.org

National Association of Social Workers (NASW)
750 First Street NE, Suite 700
Washington, DC 20002
(800) 742-4089
credentialing@naswdc.org
www.naswdc.org

The National Certification Commission for Acupuncture and Oriental Medicine (NCCAOM)
26 South Laura Street
Jacksonville, FL 32202
(904) 598-5001
www.nccaom.org

National Vulvodynia Association (NVA)
PO Box 4491
Silver Springs, MD 20914
(301) 299-0775
www.nva.org

North American Menopause Society (NAMS)
5900 Landerbrook Drive, Suite 390
Mayfield Heights, OH 44124
(440) 442-7550
www.menopause.org

Overlapping Conditions Alliance (OCA)
www.endwomenspain.org

Reflexology Association of America
PO Box 714
Chepachet, RI 02814
(980) 234-0159
www.reflexology-usa.org

Sexual Medicine Society of North America
www.smsna.org

COMPOUNDING PHARMACIES

A compounding pharmacist is expert in the preparation of medicines that are customized to meet the needs of specific situations and that are not available from pharmaceutical manufacturers.

Pharmacy Compounding Accreditation Board
www.pcab.info

Cape Drugs
384 Cape Saint Claire Road
Annapolis, MD 21401
(410) 757-3522

College Pharmacy
3505 Austin Bluffs Parkway
Colorado Springs, CO 80918
(800) 888-9358
www.collegepharmacy.com

Prescription Headquarters
1850 Front Street
East Meadow, NY 11554
(516) 222-0778
www.prescriptionheadquarters.net

Women's International Pharmacy
2 Marsh Court
Madison, WI 53718
(608) 221-7800
www.womensinternational.com

DILATORS, LUBRICANTS, AND OTHER SEXUAL AIDS

These companies have a specific understanding of sexual pain, and focus on sexual aids (like vaginal dilators and nonirritating lubricants) that help to alleviate it.

For vaginal dilators:

Overcoming Sexual Pain
www.vaginismus.com

Syracuse Medical Devices
syrmed@twcny.rr.com
(315) 449-0657

For a wide selection of lubricants, books on tantric sex, items to use as dilators, and resources for sexual aids for people with disabilities:

Proprietrix
www.grandopening.com
kim@grandopening.com

PAIN ASSESSMENT TOOLS

Measuring and Tracking Pain
www.partnersagainstpain.com/index.aspx

Numerical Pain Scale and Vulvar Pain Scale
www.healingpainfulsex.com

PELVIC FLOOR PHYSICAL THERAPISTS

The International Pelvic Pain Society
www.pelvicpain.org/providers/find-provider.aspx

Beyond Basics Physical Therapy
1560 Broadway
New York, NY 10036
(212) 354-2622
www.beyondbasicsphysicaltherapy.com

Coredynamics Physical Therapy
177 North Dean Street
Englewood, NJ 07631
(201) 568-5060
www.coredynamicspt.com

Herman & Wallace Inc.
228 Park Avenue S #71393
New York, NY 10003
(206) 724-7888
www.hermanwallace.com

5 Point Physical Therapy PLLC
596 Broadway, Suite 302
New York, NY 10012
(212) 226-2066
www.5pointpt.com

ABOUT THE AUTHORS

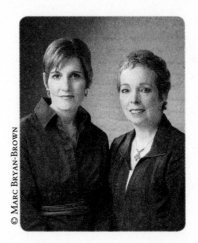

A Fellow of the American College of Obstetrics and Gynecology, Deborah Coady, MD, has been board-certified by the American Board of Obstetrics and Gynecology since 1986. She is a fellow of the New York Academy of Medicine and a member of the International Pelvic Pain Society, and has been credentialed by the North American Menopause Society as a Menopause Practitioner. In September 2009, Dr. Coady was granted a prestigious fellowship by the International Society for the Study of Vulvovaginal Disease for presenting her clinical research on vulvodynia.

In 1990, she and Dena Harris, MD, created SoHo OB/GYN, a women's healthcare center in New York City. Dr. Coady is a clinical assistant professor of Obstetrics and Gynecology at New York University Langone Medical Center. For the past two decades, she has focused the major portion of her private practice on caring for women with chronic vulvar and pelvic pain disorders.

Nancy Fish, MSW, MPH, is a licensed certified social worker with a master's degree in public health. She became a member of the National Association of Social Workers and began her private psychotherapy practice in Fair Lawn, New Jersey, in 1998. Her clinical practice has included clients requiring treatment for depression, anxiety, and anger management, and she has also provided grief counseling. Ms. Fish's approach to her clients' problems is eclectic, combining psychodymanic, cognitive-behavioral, and family life cycle therapy with particular emphasis on the relationship between the individual and herself as therapist. She specializes in helping individuals deal with chronic illness, and having experienced the impact of health crises in her own life, she brings to her work a special firsthand understanding of the challenges these patients face.

ACKNOWLEDGMENTS

THIS BOOK COULD never have been written without the help, expertise, and guidance of so many wonderful individuals. We are grateful to Rachel Kranz for her creativity and insight. Rachel, thank you from the bottom of our hearts for your outstanding editing ideas, help in making all of the medical information more accessible for the lay reader, and dedication to this essential undertaking. We are also indebted to Tracy Brown, our literary agent, for his continuous support and belief in us and in our ideas. Tracy's literary instincts and revolutionary thinking were essential in getting our book published. We also want to extend our thanks to Janis Vallely, who helped connect us to Rachel.

Thank you to Brooke Warner and Krista Lyons, our editors at Seal Press, for their unwavering support and outstanding editorial capabilities. Brooke and Krista's belief in our mission was crucial in bringing this book to publication.

We also express our deep gratitude to all our patients and their partners who so generously shared their time, personal experiences, and intimate details of their lives. Without their courage and determination, and great encouragement, we would never have been able to write this book. We thank all of you for your heroic acts of openness and kindness.

We received guidance, encouragement, and input from many of our colleagues in medicine who devotedly care for women with chronic pelvic and vulvar pain, and would like to extend our deepest appreciation to them all. A tremendous thanks to: Grace Bandow, MD; Miriam Biddleman, MSW; Struan Coleman, MD, PhD; A. Lee Dellon, MD, PhD; Eden Fromberg, DO; Stacey Futterman, PT; Dena Harris, MD; Niva Herzig, PT; Heather

Howard, MBA, PhD; Susan Kellog-Spadt, CRNP, PhD; Hollis Potter, MD; Jessica Robertson-Papp, MD; Tamer Seckin, MD; Roberta Shapiro, DO; Amy Stein, PT; Nadya Swedan, MD; and Kristene Whitmore, MD.

A special thanks to our illustrator, Arielle Marks, for his great artistry, originality, and patience with us. We also want to thank Deborah's daughter, Michelle Goodman, whose knowledge, creativity, and technical skills helped us so much.

Nancy wants to thank her husband and children—Larry, Ilona, Amy, and Scott—her sister, Irene, and her close friends: You all demonstrated extraordinary patience, provided essential emotional support, and believed wholeheartedly in the importance of our work. I am so grateful to you for being such amazing cheerleaders throughout the years of writing this book.

Deborah devotes this book to her long-term partner in medical practice, Dena Harris, MD. Dena, without you, and your patience and hard work, I could never have done this. Thank you for taking such good care of our patients and practice while I was writing and recovering from my year-long illness—all without a word of complaint. I am forever in your debt. I also want to thank my husband, Mick, and my children, Coady and Michelle, who supported me despite my frequent distractions from their lives during this long process. Thank you for helping me fulfill my dream of writing this book. I love you so much.

INDEX

· · · · · · · · · ·

Self, D or penis

genito femoral, 187
ilioinguinal
iliohypogastric

SELECTED TITLES FROM SEAL PRESS

For more than thirty years, Seal Press has published groundbreaking books.
By women. For women.

What You Really Really Want: The Smart Girl's Shame-Free Guide to Sex and Safety, by Jaclyn Friedman. $17.00, 978-1-58005-344-0. An educational and interactive guide that gives young women the tools they need to decipher the modern world's confusing, hypersexualized landscape and define their own sexual identity.

Naked at Our Age: Talking Out Loud About Senior Sex, by Joan Price. $16.95, 978-1-58005-338-9. Full of information from doctors, social workers, psychologists, and sex experts, this is an indispensable guide to handling and understanding the issues seniors face when it comes to relationships and sex.

Sexier Sex: Lessons from the Brave New Sexual Frontier, by Regina Lynn. $14.95, 978-1-58005-231-3. A fun, provocative guide to discovering your sexuality and getting more pleasure from your sensual life.

Sexual Intimacy for Women: A Guide for Same-Sex Couples, by Glenda Corwin, Ph.D. $16.95, 978-1-58005-303-7. In this prescriptive and poignant book, Glenda Corwin, PhD, helps female couples overcome obstacles to sexual intimacy through her examination of the emotional, physical, and psychological aspects of same-sex relationships.

Invisible Girls: The Truth about Sexual Abuse, by Dr. Patti Feuereisen with Caroline Pincus. $16.95, 978-1-58005-301-3. An important book for teenage girls, young women, and those who care about them, that gives hope and encouragement to sexual abuse survivors by letting them know that they're not alone and that there are many roads to healing.

The Purity Myth: How America's Obsession with Virginity Is Hurting Young Women, by Jessica Valenti. $16.95, 978-1-58005-314-3. With her usual balance of intelligence and wit, Valenti presents a powerful argument that girls and women, even in this day and age, are overly valued for their sexuality—and that this needs to stop.

FIND SEAL PRESS ONLINE
www.SealPress.com
www.Facebook.com/SealPress